the NURSE MANAGER'S GUIDE to HIRING, FIRING & INSPIRING

Vicki Hess, MS, RN, CSP

Sigma Theta Tau International
Honor Society of Nursing®

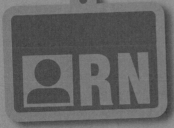

Sigma Theta Tau International

Sigma Theta Tau International
550 West North Street
Indianapolis, IN 46202

To order additional books, buy in bulk, or order for corporate use, contact Nursing Knowledge International at 888.NKI.4YOU (888.654.4968/US and Canada) or +1.317.634.8171 (outside US and Canada).

To request a review copy for course adoption, e-mail solutions@nursingknowledge.org or call 888.NKI.4YOU (888.654.4968/US and Canada) or +1.317.917.4983 (outside US and Canada).

To request author information, or for speaker or other media requests, contact Rachael McLaughlin of the Honor Society of Nursing, Sigma Theta Tau International at 888.634.7575 (US and Canada) or +1.317.634.8171 (outside US and Canada).

ISBN-13: 978-1-930538-92-4

Library of Congress Cataloging-in-Publication Data

Hess, Vicki , 1959-
  The nurse manager's guide to hiring, firing, and inspiring / Vicki Hess.
     p. ; cm.
Includes bibliographical references and index.
ISBN 978-1-930538-92-4
1. Nurse administrators. I. Sigma Theta Tau International. II. Title.

[DNLM: 1. Nurses--organization & administration. 2. Personnel Management--methods. 3. Motivation. WY 30 H586n 2010]
  RT89.3.H47 2010
  362.17'3068--dc22
                          2010010836

First Printing, 2010

Publisher: Renee Wilmeth

Acquisitions Editor: Cynthia Saver, RN, MS

Development Editor: John Sleeva

Copy Editor: Brian Walls

Cover Designer: Katy Bodenmiller

Principal Editor: Carla Hall

Editorial Coordinator: Paula Jeffers

Proofreader: Barbara Bennett

Indexer: Jane Palmer

Illustrations, Interior Design, and Page Composition: Studio Galou

Dedication

This book is dedicated with heartfelt thanks to every nurse who ever taught me, worked with me, or cared for me. Especially to Mary Heckel, RN, and Bunny Kohn, RN, whose tender loving care made a very trying experience bearable.

Acknowledgements

A community is a group of people who support each other through thick and thin. These days, the great thing about community is that we can connect virtually or face-to-face every day. Regardless of the frequency of our time together, I would like to offer my sincere thanks to my community of family, friends, and colleagues who helped me in writing this book.

First, I want to thank my family for their support. Cindi Fielder, you are a great sounding board and contributor. Josh, you artfully helped with survey results and shared your citation expertise so that all of the credit was given when due. Brian, you made life easy by doing so well at school. Alan, you laughed with me, supported me, and loved me through the process (again).

Susan Bindon and Joy Goldman, you are constant supporters who offered your talent and brain power when I got stuck. Thank you for helping me to see things in a new light on more than one occasion.

Lee Cook, I appreciate how generously you shared your time and talents in researching topics with me.

Thank you to Bill Moore, Denise Rouse-Meekins, Patricia Hart, and Stephanie Reid for helping me set up focus groups, and to all of the focus-group participants for sharing your insights with me.

I appreciate the time that almost 300 friends and strangers took to complete my on-line questionnaire. Pam Young, thank you for helping me to understand the nuances of using the survey narrative in my writing. Your insights were illuminating.

Juli Baldwin, I can hear your voice in my mind as I write each day. You are an excellent teacher and a very good friend.

Janet Ladd, Jason Nemoy, Donna Monius, Barbara Bartels, Susan Glinsman, Bette Nunn, Valerie Zamora, Terry Bennett, Anna Gray, Dawn Morrison, and Cory Silkman—thanks for the time you took to read chapters along the way and to give your feedback.

Dr. Sam Ross, thanks for breakfast meetings to share your insights about health care today and the important role of nurse managers. Martha Lessman-Katz, I appreciate your attention to detail and great ideas as I got started.

Renee Wilmeth, Cindy Saver, Carla Hall, Louisa Adair, and all the Sigma Theta Tau International and Nursing Knowledge International folks, I appreciate your support and guidance during this process.

Finally, I'd like to give a shout out to Kathy Pagana who got this whole party started. Thanks, Kathy, for thinking of me and for being such a great mentor, friend, and NSA buddy!

Thank you, community, from the bottom of my heart.

About the Author

Vicki Hess, RN, MS, CSP, is the founder and principal of Catalyst Consulting, LLC. A highly-regarded speaker, author, facilitator, and consultant, Hess is an expert in employee engagement, team dynamics, and workforce and leadership development with more than 25 years of hands-on business experience. Prior to starting her company in 2001, she was responsible for nonclinical employee training, team building, customer service, and leadership development for 6,000 employees at LifeBridge Health. Earlier in her career, Hess was in major account sales for Xerox Corporation and managed a training department for a major computer retailer. A registered nurse, she also has more than a decade of experience in the health care industry.

Hess is a certified speaking professional (CSP), the speaking profession's international standard for platform skill. Fewer than 10 percent of all professional speakers worldwide have completed the five-year process for CSP designation by the National Speakers Association. She holds a master's degree in human resource development from Towson University and was an adjunct professor at the Johns Hopkins University Graduate School of Business for five years where she taught Principles of Training and Development.

Hess's professional experiences and original workplace research led her to develop her proprietary **Professional Paradise**™ concept and proven *SHIFT*™ methodology for permanently changing unproductive thought patterns, actions, and habits. When life threw her a sucker punch in 2008 and she was diagnosed with stage one ovarian cancer, she used her own strategies and techniques to prove that people can *shift* and find authentic joy at work and in life, no matter what comes their way. (After surgery and chemotherapy, Hess's prognosis is now excellent.)

Hess is the author of *SHIFT to Professional Paradise: 5 Steps to Less Stress, More Energy & Remarkable Results at Work* and the *28-Day Diary Series*™—a collection of innovative workbooks that transform readers through long-term habit change. She is also a regular contributor to the *Baltimore Business Journal*.

Hess's husband, two almost-grown sons, and dog, Gabby, are the source of much of her joy and humor.

Table of Contents

Introduction

A Nurse Manager's Partial Daily To-Do List

- Improve patient safety
- Improve patient satisfaction
- Improve employee engagement
- Create and manage the budget while lowering expenses
- Decrease errors and "never events"
- Hire new staff
- Conduct performance appraisals
- Discipline staff
- Stay on top of clinical advances
- Learn new technology
- Conduct meetings
- Attend meetings

Most people would get tired just reading this partial list of responsibilities that you hold as a nurse manager. Many managers from outside of health care would wonder in amazement and ask, "How do you do it?" Some nurse managers wonder how to get it done, and I'm here to help.

Are you ready for real-world strategies for real managers with real to-do lists? My intention in this book is to share strategies that are practical, tactical, and implementable in the midst of the everyday challenges you face as a nurse manager. I translate current research and combine it with actual stories and years of experience to help you create a new reality that includes having the right person in the right job doing the right work—in other words, a team of highly engaged employees. Because when it comes to providing health care today, this is where the rubber meets the road. Your responsibility is vast, the pressures are real, and the rewards abound. Now is the time, today is the day, and this is one of the tools to help you on your journey.

When I first thought about writing this book, I must admit that I was nervous. I have never been a nurse manager, so I was afraid I would not be able to help you, the nurse manager, in your quest to be excellent at what you do. What I found was that the wisdom gleaned from my years as a staff nurse and training manager, my time spent working with thousands of nurses and nurse managers in the education department for a multi-facility health system and in my consulting practice, and my master's degree in human resources provided an ideal foundation—but I still felt like I needed more. I wanted to hear from actively practicing nurses and their managers, both in writing and in person.

So, I got busy. I created an online questionnaire and sent it to everyone I knew across the U.S. with an invitation to share the link with all the nurses they knew. Through six degrees of separation and social networking, I ended up with 200 nurses and 85 nurse managers completing the survey. I never set out to re-create comprehensive research that has been completed by organizations such as Gallup or the Conference Board. That research is sound and quoted in this book. Instead, I wanted to hear, in the nurses' own words, the ups and downs of working for and being a nurse manager in an ever-changing health care environment. Once the surveys started coming in, I expanded the dialogue through focus groups.

Thanks to the time and insights volunteered by the wonderful nurses and nurse managers from Carroll County Hospital Center in Westminster, Maryland, Sinai Hospital of Baltimore, Maryland, St Joseph Medical Center in South Bend, Indiana, and Atlanta Medical Center, Atlanta Georgia, I was able to expand the dialogue. These nurse managers and nurses provided more depth and richness through their open and honest dialogue about their jobs. I also conducted telephone interviews with other nurse managers, nurse recruiters, and health care human resources professionals as well as informal meetings with nurse educators and nurse managers to expand the conversation.

As a result of these conversations, I decided to organize the book as follows:

- **Part I—Hiring SMARTT:** You can't possibly meet your departmental goals without having the right players on the team doing what they are supposed to be doing. That's where Hiring SMARTT comes in. If you take the time to hire the correct person for the job, then the job of inspiring is much easier. In our first job we all learned as we watched our boss and co-workers that some people work harder, some people have a better attitude, and some people are a better fit. Most of us are drawn to those properly hired people whether they are co-workers, bosses, or others we encounter at work because they are satisfied, energized, and productive. The six steps of Hiring SMARTT provide the tools for hiring and are critical to your long-term success as a manager.

- **Part II—The Inspiring Manager:** When it comes to inspiring employees, the job gets a little trickier. Differences in employees and what motivates them provide you with opportunities to grow your employee engagement skills. In the second section, I outline and explain the Partnership Protocol™, a model with five elements that acts as a roadmap for engaging others on the job. Additionally, I share the components of the Performance Platform™, a foundational tool for managing staff performance.

- **Part III—Resignations and Firings:** The last component of the book relates to voluntary or involuntary separation. Relationships between an employee and employer come to an end. Whether you are initiating the change or the employee has chosen to leave, important factors to help you are included in this section of the book.

Each chapter offers practical advice from experienced nurse managers, a variety of sources, and my own experience. The vignettes I share are not based on any one person; they are a compilation of my experiences, comments from the questionnaire, and my observations from working with my healthcare clients. Any direct quotes from the survey are referenced and are anonymous—even to me.

In some sections I paraphrase, in the most accurate way possible, the thoughts that were shared in the focus groups. Together, this mixed approach adds volumes to the research done by others and sets out to provide you with just the right strategies you need for tackling the everyday struggles and successes associated with hiring, firing, and inspiring staff.

In addition to real-life examples, I share various tools, models, and specific suggestionsto help you feel more proactive and less reactive in your work as a nurse manager. You'll see many boxes throughout the text with examples, stories, homework, and helpful hints. The book is written in an easily digestible manner because I know you already have a lot to do. The aim is to make your job easier, not more complicated.

Most importantly, my intention is to be of service to you so that you can be of service to the frontline caregivers. Together, we all make a difference in the lives of those who need health care. As the nation's politicians, scholars, shareholders, and health care providers wrestle with how to manage health care in the upcoming years, we know that nurses (and therefore nurse managers) will always be a part of the equation. As you go about your days and engage in hiring, inspiring, and yes, maybe even firing staff, I wish you a journey full of smooth roads, great friendships, and most importantly, healing for all.

–Vicki Hess, RN, MS, CSP

PART I

Hiring SMARTT

Imagine your department fully staffed—all the employees get along and support each other, the patients appreciate the great care and service, the physicians are happy and helpful, other departments are cooperative and ready to lend a hand, and the organization's leadership uses your department as an example for all to see. Have I lost you in a fit of laughter … or tears … or can you picture it?

When you Hire SMARTT, you lay the foundation for creating the environment I just described. When you Hire SMARTT, you find the right person for the right job—as well as someone who is energized, satisfied, and productive. Hiring SMARTT allows for highly engaged employees, outstanding organizational results, and a great fit for all employees.

Hiring SMARTT involves the following six steps:

- **S**tart with strengths in mind.
- **M**ake a list of behavior-based questions.
- **A**sk questions and listen carefully.
- **R**eview responses and compare candidates.
- **T**ake your time and make the hiring decision.
- **T**houghtfully bring the new person on board.

Hiring SMARTT involves finding the person with the right strengths to fill the open position. The second part of the hiring equation is creating a strategic connection. You should be thinking about this connection early in the hiring process. From the very first interview, you want to share the strategic value that the ope position has within the organization.

CHAPTER 1
Start with Strengths in Mind

Hiring SMARTT

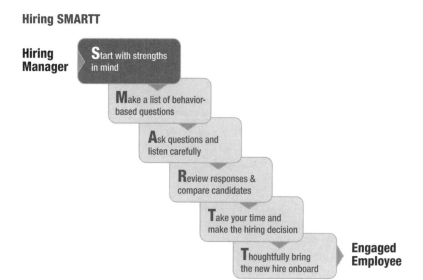

If you want to hire the right person—the person who really fits your department and the position you have open—start with the end in mind. Being specific about the result you desire creates clarity that will pay tenfold during the hiring process. When you find someone with the strengths you need, you have found an A+ Candidate.

Don't worry, I am not asking you to become a human resources expert with in-depth knowledge of writing competency statements or detailed job descriptions (although this is often helpful in the long run). I am simply asking you to identify and prioritize the key behaviors—the strengths—you would like the A+ Candidate to consistently demonstrate.

The following sections discuss the four steps to complete this process:

1. Create an initial list of desired strengths.
2. Identify your top performers' strengths.
3. Identify overlap between #1 and #2.
4. Create a final list of strengths.

Creating an Initial List of Desired Strengths

I encourage you to find some quiet time (I know this might have some of you chuckling, but give it a try) to think about the strengths you are looking for in an A+ Candidate. Think about the top performers on your team. What strengths do they possess that you would like to see more of? Or, what strengths are missing that you would like to find? Do not focus on personality traits; instead, focus on strengths that they bring to the job through their behaviors.

Behaviors fall into two broad categories: *clinical strengths* and *performance strengths*. Most nurse managers seem to find it easier to identify clinical strengths than to identify performance strengths. You may think you can skip this step because you know these clinical and performance strengths intuitively, but I strongly encourage you to take the time. This step adds clarity to the interviewing process as it requires careful consideration. If you skip this step, later steps will be more difficult.

Clinical strengths are the technical skills needed in your area of nursing. For example, if you are hiring a postpartum nurse, your list might include the following clinical strengths (in no particular order):

- Newborn assessment skills
- Breastfeeding education
- Routine care of postpartum patients
- Caring for post-surgical patients

You cannot possibly make a list of *all* clinical strengths, so focus on the specific skills that are most important for your area.

Performance strengths are those nonclinical behaviors that A+ Candidates demonstrate that lead to the smooth operation of the unit or department. Again, it is helpful to think of the top performers on your team when creating this list. Examples of performance strengths include the following:

- Working well in a team
- Patient satisfaction skills
- Effective use of technology
- Leadership skills

When you are identifying the desired performance strengths, think about nature versus nurture. Which strengths or skills need to be part of someone's internal make-up (nature) and which strengths can you teach them (nurture)? Most managers would agree that it is much easier to teach someone to use hospital-specific technology than it is to teach someone to be nice to their patients. During the hiring process, ensure that the candidate possesses the desired internal strengths (nature) so that your time is spent training them on the teachable skills that are not part of their DNA.

Collecting Your Top Performers' Lists of Strengths

Remeber your top performers from Step 1? Well ask them to write down 8–10 strengths they would like a new co-worker to possess. Do not be too prescriptive or define parameters; your goal is to get your top performers' original thoughts, not what they think you might want them to say. These objective perspectives are very helpful when creating the final A+ Candidate list.

Identifying List Overlap

This step is fairly straightforward. Compare your list with the lists you receive from the top performers, noting where the lists overlap.

Most nurse managers will see a trend of ideal strengths; these ideal strengths will provide the basis for Step 4.

Creating a Final List of Strengths

When you can clearly identify the trends from the lists you review, decide which 5–7 key clinical, performance, culture, and team strengths constitute an A+ Candidate for your area. This list will be a barometer against which you will measure candidates during the interview process. Keep this list of A+ Candidate strengths handy, because you will need it as we progress to the next step. The following is an abbreviated version of what your list might look like for a unit secretary.

Clinical Strengths (Technical skills needed for job)

1. Knowledge of medical terminology
2. Adept at computer usage

Performance Strengths (Nonclinical behaviors that top candidates demonstrate on the job)

1. Strong attention to detail
2. Able to juggle multiple tasks simultaneously

Organizational/Culture Strengths (Behaviors that create fit within the organization overall)

1. Enjoys fast-paced environment
2. Seeks out learning opportunities

Team Strengths (Skills & behaviors that add to effective team work in department)

1. Positive attitude towards others
2. Offers to help before being asked

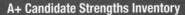

Time-Saver Tools

A+ Candidate Strengths Inventory

Take a shortcut in creating your A+ Candidate strengths list. Use the inventory I've created to save time.

www.HiringFiringInspiring.com

Don't Reinvent the Wheel

Betsy, a nurse manager at a community teaching hospital, worked with other nurse managers in her specialty—critical-care—to create a list of performance strengths for nurses in that area. She started with the American Association of Critical-Care Nurses (AACN) Standards for Establishing and Sustaining Healthy Work Environments (2005). The standards include skilled communication, true collaboration, effective decision making, appropriate staffing, meaningful recognition, and authentic leadership. Of this list, the first three standards relate to staff nursing and were included on the strengths list that Betsy created. The information from AACN, providing detail about what these phrases mean, was very helpful for Betsy.

Remember, you do not have to start from scratch. Use what is available and accurate.

Summary

When beginning the process of hiring someone, keep in mind the strengths that you are looking for. Identify which strengths are most important to you and your team through the following steps:

1. Create your list of desired strengths.

2. Ask your top performers to list the strengths they want in a co-worker.

3. Find the overlap.

4. Make the final list of strengths.

Whether the position is for nursing or ancillary staff, starting with strengths in mind and a clear idea of what you are looking for in a new team member helps you narrow your search, focus your training, and find the A+ Candidate for the open position.

CHAPTER 2
Make a List of Behavior-Based Questions

RN

Hiring SMARTT

Hiring Manager

Start with strengths in mind

Make a list of behavior-based questions

Ask questions and listen carefully

Review responses & compare candidates

Take your time and make the hiring decision

Thoughtfully bring the new hire onboard

Engaged Employee

Have you heard the technology expression, "garbage in, garbage out"? The premise is that if you program a computer with faulty code, the output will be faulty as well. Unfortunately, for many nurse managers, the same thing happens during the interview process. Faulty questions lead to faulty responses, which, in turn, hide potential problems with job candidates. The results are frustrating when the new hire doesn't work out in the end. The nurse manager is left thinking, "He or she seemed great in the interview – what happened?" In many cases, the nurse manager might simply be hiring from the heart. This problem can be solved with a careful examination and retooling of the questions that you ask during an interview.

I've asked hundreds of managers for their favorite interviewing questions. Here are a few of the most popular examples:

- Where do you see yourself in five years?
- Why do you want to work here?
- How will you contribute to our unit/organization?

What these questions have in common is that they are hypothetical. Unfortunately, if you ask a hypothetical question, you get a hypothetical answer. Because you aren't making a hypothetical hiring decision, you need a way to uncover *real* responses from job candidates—not *hypothetical* responses.

The best way to avoid the "garbage in, garbage out" phenomenon in hiring is to ask *behavior-based questions.*

Asking Behavior-Based Questions

Behavior-based questions ask about past behavior, not future unknowns. According to the Society for Human Resource Management (SHRM), "behavioral-based questions follow the psychological premise that past behavior predicts future performance. In other words, if an applicant has done something in the past, he or she is likely to do it again in the future" (2008). Behavioral interviewing was created by Behavioral Technology, Inc. in the 1970s to increase the effectiveness of interviewers hiring the right person for the right job.

It makes a lot of sense, doesn't it? If a health care provider has handled a situation in the past, he or she is likely to master the situation in your work environment in the future. Instead of hoping that the applicant can do the job, he or she tells you about a specific example where he or she has done it already.

Here are some of the benefits of behavior-based questioning:

- Creates a systematic approach.
- Acquires relevant and objective information.
- Provides best match between candidate and job.

- Reduces job turnover.
- Reduces training time.
- Protects from lawsuits.
- Improves team morale.

A few standard sentence starters easily create behavior-based questions for clinical skills, performance skills, organizational fit, team cohesion, and so on. These questions or phrases get the conversation going, and then you have an opportunity to dig deeper with a few "Tell me more…" phrases. The interview becomes a story-telling session. Here are some examples of sentence starters and how they can be used:

- Tell me about a time when you…
    - Had two patient emergencies at the same time.
    - Worked with a physician who was really annoying.
- Give me an example of…
    - How you handled a difficult family member.
    - When you encountered a procedure you weren't sure of.
- How do you currently…
    - Manage conflicts with co-workers?
    - Manage your stress at work?

This is how the conversation might flow as you tie questions together and dig deeper.

- Tell me about a time when you…
    - Made a mistake at work. How did you handle the mistake before, during, and after it occurred? What did you learn from the mistake?

Often managers ask a question out of habit or because someone else asked them the question, so they assume it was a good one. Let's go back to the favorite questions I listed in the beginning and determine what the manager was really trying to figure out.

Favorite Question	Desired Information
Where do you want to be in five years?	Motivation for future growth; the candidate's prescribed career path
Why do you want to work for us?	What the candidate is looking for in a job; what the candidate dislikes about a current job
How will you contribute to our unit?	Assessment of strengths; research and preparation for interview

If you flip the table and put the desired information on the left, rewriting the questions using the behavior-based format forces the candidate to share a past example to illustrate the point. Additionally, you receive tangible examples of what the candidate has actually done rather than vague platitudes and hypothetical musings.

Desired Information	Behavior-Based Questions
Motivation for future growth; the candidate's prescribed career path	What have you done in the past two months for professional development?
What the candidate is looking for in a job; what the candidate dislikes about a current job	When you made your last job change, what were you looking for? What do you dislike about your current job?
Assessment of strengths; research and preparation for interview	On your last performance review, what did your boss say are your strengths? How did you prepare for this interview?

Writing Questions

Think about a job that you are trying to fill. Review the list of clinical strengths and performance strengths that you created in Chapter 1. Using the table frame I've provided on the next page, select an appropriate sentence starter and write a behavior-based question for that skill area for each competency that you list.

Clinical or Performance Strength	Behavior-Based Question	Priority Ranking
Handling complex medical patients	Tell me about a time when you were responsible for handling 3-4 medically complex patients.	

Make sure the questions ask about past behavior and are not hypothetical.

After the questions are written, prioritize the related strengths by importance for the position you are trying to fill. Which ones are "nice to have" versus "need to have"? Also, think about which strengths are nature versus nurture. You can train someone to insert an IV line, but can you train someone to come to work every day with a great attitude? Often, you discover that finding a candidate who already possesses key performance strengths takes priority over finding a candidate with clinical strengths because you have the resources for teaching clinical skills in the orientation and preceptor process.

Assessing Organizational and Team Fit

Another key element is finding the right person for your organization, particularly your unit. A nurse who thrives in an academic teaching facility might find that a small community hospital lacks the challenge to which he or she is accustomed. Conversely, someone who loves the familiar family feel of a smaller patient care unit might be uncomfortable in a larger one. Like many nurse managers, you might be wondering, "How do I find out where someone best fits in a short interview?"

You guessed it! You ask behavior-based questions. Pull out your organization's mission, vision, and values statements. Determine the elements that really create the "feel" of your department and focus on these. You can also ask top performers how they would describe the culture and use their descriptions to create questions. Here are a few examples to get you started.

- Please describe the culture of the organization where you work now. What do you like or dislike about that culture?

- One of our core values is exemplary service. Give me an example in your current job that shows your commitment to providing outstanding service.

- Most people on our unit have a great sense of humor; tell me about a time where your sense of humor saved the day.

Ask for Help

In many hospitals, the nurse recruiter or HR department has already created a list of interview questions that focus on organizational fit. Starting with the culture, vision, and values, these questions can be very helpful and save you a lot of time.

Write a few questions for your culture here:

Culture Elements	Behavior-Based Question	Priority Ranking
Teaching hospital	Please share a recent example of how you mentored someone in your department.	

Asking Team Fit Questions

Effective performance requires teamwork. During the interview, you should ask a prospective employee about his or her experiences as a team player. For example:

- Tell me about a team you currently work on. What is your role?
- What strengths do you bring to the team?
- Tell me about someone you really respect on your team. What do you respect about this person?
- What frustrates you most about this team?

Take a moment to add some additional team fit questions

Team Elements	Behavior-Based Question	Priority Ranking
Offering to help	When was the last time you pitched in to help someone before being asked? Tell me about what happened.	

Time-Saver Tools
Behavior-Based Questions Prep Form

Now that you have identified the performance and clinical strengths, and elements of organizational and team fit, it's time to add the corresponding behavior-based questions so you are ready for the next step. Use this prep form to get started.

www.HiringFiringInspiring.com.

Considering Legal Issues

Another key benefit of asking behavior-based questions is that you avoid illegal interview questions. Avoid asking questions about the following:

- Disabilities
- Age
- Religion
- Family obligations
- Past arrests
- Citizenship

If you focus solely on job responsibilities and candidate capabilities, you will avoid illegal questioning.

Suppose that a job candidate is dressed in a way that reflects a religious preference and you are worried about his or her ability to work on certain days of the week. An illegal question asks about his or her religion and whether it will interfere with his or her work schedule. A legal, behavior-based question asks about the person's current work schedule. You can share the hours that you need the person to work and ask whether he or she is available to work that schedule. When in doubt, always ask someone in human resources or your legal counsel to confirm questions about which you are unsure.

Questions to Avoid

According to Falcone (2002), here are a few popular questions to avoid:

- How old are you?
- Where were you born?
- Are you married?
- Are you disabled?
- Have you ever been arrested?
- What kind of discharge did you get from the military?
- Have you ever declared bankruptcy?

These questions would give you information that could be used in a discriminatory way. Stick to behavior-based questions that focus on past behaviors and then connect the dots to the strengths you are looking for.

Summary

Before you conduct the first interview for the open position, you should have a list of behavior-based questions prepared. Rather than asking hypothetical questions, which obtain hypothetical information, ask behavior-based questions, which reflect your prospective employee's past work experience. Here's how:

- Use the list of strengths you created in Chapter 1.
- Place the recommended sentence starters before the strengths to create the behavior-based questions.
- Avoid illegal questions that relate to culture, race, age, or gender.
- Use your HR department to help you craft your questions.

Behavior-based questions enable you to cut through the hypothetical responses, delve into the candidate's past behavior and experience, and help you avoid illegal situations.

CHAPTER 3
Ask Questions and Listen Carefully

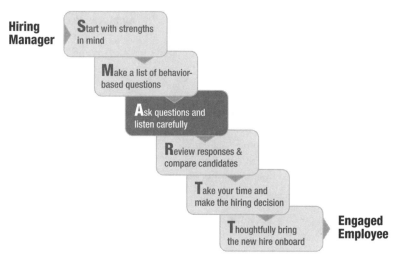

Hiring SMARTT

Hiring Manager

- **S**tart with strengths in mind
- **M**ake a list of behavior-based questions
- **A**sk questions and listen carefully
- **R**eview responses & compare candidates
- **T**ake your time and make the hiring decision
- **T**houghtfully bring the new hire onboard

Engaged Employee

Congratulations! You now have a clear list of clinical and performance strengths for the position you want to fill, as well as a comprehensive list of behavior-based questions to ask. You are officially ready for the interview. When you use the steps outlined in this chapter, you should notice a big difference in your level of confidence and control from past interviews. Remember, your goal is Hiring SMARTT.

In many organizations, a Human Resources (HR) representative initiates the interview process. A nurse recruiter or HR business partner conducts a telephone interview to prescreen the candidate. You should coordinate with the recruiter or HR rep so that he or she knows the strengths you are seeking in an A+ Candidate. When you have a smooth partnership with HR, you will feel confident that a candidate coming in for an interview is prequalified to fill the position and meets the minimum educational (and clinical) requirements.

Building Rapport

When a candidate arrives for an interview, your first responsibility is to build rapport. The idea behind building rapport is to establish trust as quickly as possible. By creating a trusting relationship early on, you encourage the job candidate to be open and honest in the interview.

To build rapport with an interviewee, start with an open-ended question that is conversational and easy to answer. For example, "How was your drive here?" or "Isn't it nice to finally see signs of spring?" Avoid questions that get too personal, such as "What are you doing over the upcoming holidays?" Keep the conversation light and comfortable to put the candidate at ease. Your job at this point is to be a gracious host.

Interviews are not a time to grill someone or make them feel like you have the upper hand (the open position). Most nurse managers understand this; however, when you are busy or feeling the stress of trying to fill a position, you might forget that you are the host of the interview and want the candidate to feel comfortable. Invite the candidate into the interviewing location, offer him or her a seat, and share your agenda for the interview.

Chatty Candidates

Watch out for the overly conversational candidate. "I'm fine. I was afraid I was going to be a few minutes late because I had to take my mother to the doctor. She had a stroke and lives with us, and I'm her primary care provider."

Your inclination might be to empathize and ask more questions, but beware. Unfortunately, even if you don't ask a question that could lead to unintentional discrimination, such as, "Are you taking care of an elderly parent?" the candidate can assert that you used the information against him or her in making your hiring decision. If the candidate starts to share information that could be construed as prejudicial, steer him or her back to the "safe zone" where you have control of the questions.

Sharing the Agenda

An interview is a business meeting, and like any well-run business meeting, you should have and share an agenda. A well-structured agenda should include the following steps:

1. Build rapport and share the day's agenda.
2. Ask behavior-based questions.
3. Discuss the open position and your unit.
4. Allow time for the candidate to ask questions.
5. Conduct a tour (only if you think there is potential for a match).
6. Discuss the next steps.

I recommend that you share the agenda with the applicant up front. Sharing the agenda might sound like this:

"Thank you for coming in today to see me, your resume looks interesting. Here's how the interview will flow. First, I will ask you a series of questions that I ask each candidate. I'll be taking notes, so don't worry if I pause to jot something down. Feel free to take notes yourself if a question comes up. Many of my questions will focus on your past work experience. I am particularly interested in hearing about past successes and challenges to figure out if you would be a good fit here in our unit. Once I am finished asking my questions, I will tell you more about the open position, and you are welcome to ask me questions about the job and its elements. Are you ready to get started?"

Remember, do not mention a tour of the facility because you might decide that this isn't a strong candidate and you don't want to feel obligated to provide one.

Asking Questions

Have your list of behavior-based questions ready on a form with space to write key elements of the response that you want to remember. Being present is a big part of making the interview work. If you are worrying about what is happening on the unit or a deadline you have to meet, you will likely miss subtle nuances, body language, or outright responses that should either raise a red flag or point out the need to ask more probing questions. Take a deep breath, relax, and start asking questions.

After you ask each question, listen to the response and read between the lines for other pertinent information. If the applicant alludes to something and you want to know more, ask a follow-up question or simply say, "Please, tell me more." The goal is not simply to ask the questions on your list; the goal is to get answers that help you make an educated selection. The more information you get during the interview, the better your hiring decision will be.

Let's Listen In

Rosa, the nurse manager in a medical unit, says, "Tell me about a time when you had two tough patients whose conditions were both deteriorating. How did you handle it?" Harris, an experienced nurse, answers, "I did the best I could. You know sometimes you just can't get to everything and you have to prioritize and some things might slip." The phrase "some things might slip" should raise a red flag. This is the time to dig deeper. Rosa should ask a probing question, such as, "Which items did you let slip?" or simply say, "Go on, and then what happened?" or my favorite, "Please tell me more."

Taking Notes

While you are asking your list of questions, you should also be taking notes. Presumably, you are interviewing several candidates for the open position, so it would be ridiculous to think that you would remember every person's responses to all your questions. Note taking often feels awkward, and we are taught to maintain eye contact when talking with someone; therefore, tell the applicant during the agenda-setting stage that you will be taking notes.

When taking notes, you should focus on objective findings, as opposed to subjective thoughts. Just like in patient care, objective data is based on fact. For example, the story of how someone handled a difficult patient is objective, whereas subjective data is your opinion about what you see or hear. "Very young and immature, seems nervous and jittery" is subjective. Both are important, but the official record of the interview should only include objective data. If you were ever called into court and asked to bring your notes, you would not want to include anything that might be assumed prejudicial. Using whatever piece of paper you have lying around and jotting down random thoughts and perceptions is not the way to go. Use a consistent format for note taking for each interview. I prefer to have the questions written down with adequate space for notes. Ask your peers and the nurse recruiter if they have a preferred method, and create your own best practices that work with your style and comfort level.

While you are listening to the applicant's responses, feel free to write down other questions that arise so that you do not inadvertently forget them. When you become more experienced asking behavior-based questions, you will realize how effective they are in uncovering practices and tendencies, which will help you determine the best fit for the open position.

To Take Notes or Not to Take Notes?

Some organizations tell managers to avoid note taking so that legal issues don't arise if they are called into court. However, done properly, note taking is a valuable tool for documentation of an interview. Imagine caring for a group of patients and not charting during your shift. Could you possibly remember the details of the care after a few shifts with a variety of patients? Most folks feel uncomfortable relying on the accuracy of their memory—and they shouldn't be asked to. The same principle applies in interviewing.

After applicants are interviewed, most managers have a tendency to remember only extremes—the really great people and the really bad folks—and the rest start to blur. The way to counteract this challenge is to take notes that focus on objective data. I mentioned earlier how helpful it is to use a simple form to record notes during the interview. Here's an example of what one might look like.

Questions	Notes	Rating
Please tell me about a time when you disagreed with a physician's order. How did you handle it? What happened?	Confidently gave 2 examples; clearly articulated the actions she took; conferred with charge nurse; called MD; asked question about order for clarification; stated that MD was angry about questions; kept calm; resolved issue; asked MD to authorize verbal order; patient given correct medication dosage; followed up with MD to get order co-signed; repaired relationship.	
Describe a team you are a part of at work now. Give me an example of a leadership role you have taken on the team.	On hand washing team. Attends meetings when she can based on work schedules – usually every other one. Stated that she doesn't really enjoy being on team and hasn't taken a leadership role at all.	

The notes act as a record of the person's response to the behavior-based question you asked and include areas where you probed more extensively. Just stick to the facts. Falcone (2002) reminds us, "The notes that you write on employee applications, resumes, or evaluation forms become part of a candidate's written record and are 'discoverable' if subpoenaed."

Time-Saver Tools
Interview Notes Form

To save time, try using this form when you interview candidates. You can also write in the questions and make copies for team interviews so you have consistency as you talk with different candidates.

www.HiringFiringInspiring.com

What's Legal to Document?

Without getting mired in legalese, it's important to understand what hiring practices might constitute discrimination. When it comes to note taking, managers are encouraged to avoid recording any comments that might lead others to believe that the candidate was discriminated against relative to the following protected classes:

- Race
- Ethnicity
- Religion
- Color
- National origin
- Age (40 and over)
- Sex
- Familial status
- Sexual orientation
- Disability status
- Veteran status

continues

- Political affiliation
- Genetic Information

The U.S. Equal Employment Opportunity Commission (EEOC), May 2009.

Be safe, never record observations about any of these areas.
Visit www.eeoc.gov for more information.

Here are a few examples of comments that could cause legal problems:

Questions	Notes	Rating
Please tell me about a time when you disagreed with a physician's order. How did you handle it? What happened?	Used "like" a lot in response; seemed kind of young and immature -sort of giggly and silly; awfully uncomfortable when trying to give examples; don't think the doctors would like her.	
Describe a team you are a part of at work now. Give me an example of a leadership role you have taken on the team.	On hand washing team; talked about working on all-female team and needing to take over because none of the women would take charge; his accent was really thick – not sure where he is from or if others would be able to understand him.	

The majority of these comments are subjective and focus on how someone answered instead of what he or she said. A sound mantra for note taking is "When in doubt, leave it out" and always check with your legal department or an HR representative if you are unsure.

Great News

Most nurse managers already possess fantastic patient assessment skills and many of these skills are transferable to assessing job candidates. According to the American Nurses Association, the nursing process is the common thread for registered nurses providing holistic, patient-centered care. The web site adds that the first step of the nursing process is assessment. During the assessment, "an RN uses a systematic, dynamic way to collect and analyze data about a client."

Using patient assessment skills to assess job candidates should be an easy transition. Just tap into your well-honed clinical assessment skills when reviewing responses and evaluate candidates based on the desired strengths you outline.

Digging Deeper

One of the hazards of using behavior-based questions is that responses often require careful thinking, which takes time. If the applicant stumbles or an awkward silence ensues, say something like, "It's okay if it takes you a minute to think of an answer. I know these questions can be tough." You can think about your next question or make notes on other responses. Don't accept artificial answers for the sake of avoiding the awkward silence. Probe the applicant and be patient until you get enough information to satisfy your well-honed clinical assessment skills.

Another common practice of experienced interviewers is to seek contrary evidence—that is, information that goes against the grain of what you are hearing. For example, Calvin, a prospective ER nurse, is responding to questions about how he has handled high-pressure situations in the past. He seems to be a super hero and has detailed responses for your toughest questions about managing his stress on the job. You are beginning to wonder if anyone can be this good. (Secretly you hope he is and that he will come to work for you.) This is the time to seek contrary evidence. The conversation might include, "Calvin, you have given me several strong examples of how you have handled the stress of working in a busy ER. Please tell me about a time when you did not cope as well and things fell apart." Give him a chance to think of something that is contrary to the picture that he has been painting. Avoid the temptation of taking responses at face value and dig deeper.

Take Time to Practice

The best way to get good at anything is to practice. Take time to set up a mock interview with another nurse manager or a nurse recruiter. You can take turns asking each other questions, taking notes, and digging deeper. Be realistic in your responses when you are role-playing as the job candidate. This realism will help you immensely when the actual interview takes place.

Conducting Group Interviews

Sometimes it is a good idea to have more than one interviewer at a time and conduct a group interview. Several reasons you might want to conduct a group interview include:

- To create buy-in from current staff for the selection process.

- To account for time constraints for the interviews (especially if an applicant is from out of town) or if interviewers have a tight schedule.

- To assess how someone handles the pressure of a group setting.

Before conducting a group interview, however, I recommend that you conduct a one-on-one interview to get to know the candidate and to ease the person into the behavior-based questioning process. When the group interview occurs (you could have anywhere from 2–6 people present), predetermine the questions to ask, put them on a form, and give everyone a copy. Assign everyone a few questions and instruct them to take objective notes. Before the interview starts, review the characteristics of the A+ Candidate that you determined in the first step of Hiring SMARTT (refer to Chapter 1). This reminder about strengths you are seeking helps you avoid the "gut feeling" barometer that many inexperienced interviewers use.

Share Days

Almost every nurse manager I speak with sings the praises of having a "share day" for any prospective hire. Assuming the candidate has met the prescreening requirements of HR and passed muster at your one-on-one interview (and the group interview, if one was held), it's time for a share day. Invite the candidate to spend at least 4 hours in your department shadowing one of your top performers.

The visiting candidate will not be providing direct patient care, but will have a chance to experience a typical day in your department. The staff member who is being shadowed will also have a chance to get to know the candidate and ask more questions. Some managers split the time spent in the department between two experienced nurses to provide different viewpoints for all involved. Be sure to schedule time to meet with the candidate before the day is over to see what he or she thought and answer any questions. Only invite someone to a share day if you think he or she is a good fit.

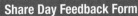

Time-Saver Tools

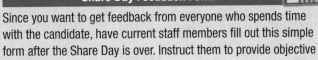

Share Day Feedback Form

Since you want to get feedback from everyone who spends time with the candidate, have current staff members fill out this simple form after the Share Day is over. Instruct them to provide objective feedback.

www.HiringFiringInspiring.com

Privacy Warning

Talk with the nurse recruiter and HR about any release or confidentiality forms that need to be signed prior to an interviewee spending time with patients. Make sure the candidate knows the confidential nature of his or her interactions with patients.

Summary

To maximize the time you spend in the process of interviewing, create a consistent structure by performing the following steps:

1. Establish rapport with small talk to put the candidate at ease and begin to build trust.

2. Share the agenda for the interview and maintain control during the process by following the agenda.

3. Ask the questions you developed with your HR department earlier to uncover the information you are looking for. Take your time and allow the candidate to take a few moments to answer each question thoughtfully.

4. Make sure you listen very carefully to your candidate and dig deeper by probing and seeking contrary evidence when appropriate.

5. Have your mind on the interview and not elsewhere, or you might miss an informative aspect of the interview.

6. Take structured notes that are objective rather then scribbling on a loose page.

By following these steps, you will be on your way to hiring the candidate you desire.

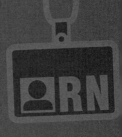

CHAPTER 4
Review Responses and Evaluate Candidates

Hiring SMARTT

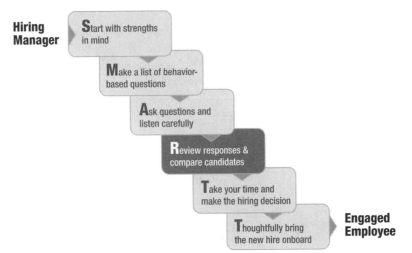

Hiring Manager

Start with strengths in mind

Make a list of behavior-based questions

Ask questions and listen carefully

Review responses & compare candidates

Take your time and make the hiring decision

Thoughtfully bring the new hire onboard

Engaged Employee

The interview process is moving along. You started with strengths in mind, made your list of behavior-based questions, and then asked questions and listened carefully. Now you are ready to review the responses and evaluate candidates. If you have taken good notes, the review process should be straightforward. When evaluating candidates, you should focus on how well the person compares to the strengths you listed in Chapter 1. The goal, as many nurse managers have shared, is finding the right fit.

A challenge in the candidate review phase is sorting through fact versus perception. As with patient care, your assessment should be twofold:

- **Observational:** Pay attention to subtle nuances, body language, and inconsistencies in responses. For example, if the interviewee starts to blush, lacks eye contact, or wiggles around in his or her seat, these might be indications of discomfort on his or her part. Without being an expert in body language, you can still pay attention to what seems appropriate for the questions being asked.

- **Evidence-based:** Focus on actual details from someone's past experience. Review the responses you noted during the interview and look for trends. For example, if the interviewee mentions ways he or she deals with stress in a productive manner in response to more than one question, it most likely indicates a pattern that will be repeated in the future.

A second challenge is remembering each candidate during the process. Taking good notes is critical for both elements (as discussed in Chapter 3).

Shopping for Applicants

Avoid the temptation of comparing one candidate to another right away. You might end up with the best of the mediocre. Imagine that you are at the grocery store buying apples for a pie. All the apples are brown and mushy. In the absence of fresh apples, you might think about comparing a few oranges, plums, and peaches to see which ones look freshest; however, in the end it doesn't matter because you need fresh apples for your pie recipe.

When evaluating candidates, keep the end in mind, pull out your list of desired strengths, and proceed from there. Stick to your list because in this case, a peach pie just won't do!

The Rating Scale

An important tool to help you make a sound hiring decision is the rating scale. Although many varieties of rating scales exist, the most important aspect of any scale is your consistency in using it. The purpose of the rating scale is to help you compare the applicants to strengths you seek and, ultimately, to each other. The following is an example of rating criteria I recommend:

5. **Role model:** Applicant shares examples of exemplary performance in this area. He or she has proven track record as evidenced by extensive knowledge, certification, and comfort with the topic.

4. **Competent:** Applicant shares examples of routine performance in this area. He or she is able to independently perform the skills.

3. **Needs some development:** Applicant requires assistance in completing the skills. Examples highlight the need for continued development in this area.

2. **Needs extensive development:** Applicant has only occasionally demonstrated this skill either because of lack of opportunity or lack of knowledge or ability. Significant resources are needed to be competent.

1. **Novice:** Applicant has never demonstrated this strength and needs to learn the skills associated with it.

Your HR department may have a scale they prefer, and that's fine as well. Just remember that each interviewer should use the same scale with each candidate. Consistency is key at this point in your decision-making process.

One reason I recommend the preceding rating scale is that it is user-friendly. The descriptive words could be used by anyone without extensive training. Based on the definitions, everyone can easily agree on what is deemed as a role model, competent, novice, and so on.

When the interview is over and the candidate has gone, spend a few minutes to review your notes and rate each response using the scale (see the following table). You can total the scores and give the person an average. Ask each person who interviews the candidate to use the same scale—you'll have more data to consider, helping you find the best fit for the open position.

Questions	Notes	Rating
Please tell me about a time when you disagreed with a physician's order. How did you handle it? What happened?	Confidently gave 2 examples; clearly articulated the actions she took; conferred with charge nurse; called MD; asked question about order for clarification; stated that MD was angry about questions; kept calm; resolved issue; asked MD to authorize verbal order; patient given correct medication dosage; followed up with MD to get order co-signed; repaired relationship.	5. Role model
Describe a team you are a part of at work now. Give me an example of a leadership role you have taken on the team.	On hand-washing team; attends meetings when she can, based on work schedules—usually every other one; stated that she doesn't really enjoy being on team and hasn't taken a leadership role at all.	2. Needs extensive development

Buyer Beware

When rating applicants, be as objective as possible. Unfortunately, we humans make decisions about others that might include biases. The first step towards objectivity is to be aware of potential biases we each have. We all bring beliefs and mind-sets to work that color our impressions of others. Just because you have these beliefs and mind-sets, doesn't mean you have to act upon them.

Examples of errors raters may make include:

- **Bias:** Bringing personal feelings or prejudices into the process.
- **Halo effect:** Viewing performance as all good or all bad.
- **Central tendency:** Giving all candidates a medium rating.

- **Similar-to-me:** Giving more favorable ratings to people who are more characteristically like you.
- **Stereotyping:** Applying generalizations (based on race, gender, nationality, etc.).

http://www.hr.eku.edu/development/performance/resources.php#errors

Prehire Testing

Another tool in your toolbox when it comes to Hiring SMARTT, and specifically reviewing and evaluating candidates, is preemployment testing. Many preemployment testing options are available to nurse managers today. The Association of Test Publishers, as reported in www.etesting.com, states, "Professionally developed tests that are designed by experts, and scored and interpreted by properly trained individuals, can help even the most experienced and knowledgeable decision-maker to construct a fairer and more accurate picture of an individual."

According to the U. S. Equal Employment Opportunity Commission (EEOC), the following tests are acceptable as long as they do not discriminate against any of the protected classes outlined in Chapter 3:

- Cognitive tests
- Physical ability tests
- Sample job tasks
- Medical inquiries and physical examinations
- Personality tests and integrity tests
- Criminal background checks
- Credit checks
- English proficiency tests

www.eeoc.gov, 2009

Talk with the nurse recruiter or an HR representative to see what your organization's policy is regarding testing, including what instruments are commonly used for hiring patient care staff.

Typically, nurse managers do not need to select or administer preemployment tests. HR usually handles this, and the nurse manager receives only candidates who have passed the minimum requirements. This is another example of where a strong relationship with the recruiter will help you find the best candidate for your open position.

References

The majority of nurse managers I spoke with stated that HR professionals or nurse recruiters check references. Usually, candidates are asked to fill out a consent form that allows the organization to contact references. Unfortunately, despite this permission-based system, current and former employers are often reluctant to talk about job candidates because of worries about potential lawsuits. Getting solid information when checking references is a multi-step process, and because HR typically makes the calls, I will not review it here.

The bottom line is that reference checks are another weapon in your Hiring SMARTT arsenal. Up to this point, your opinion of the candidate is based solely on your interaction with him or her. It makes sense to hear a former supervisor's opinion as well. Proactively ask HR for the information they gathered during reference checks so that you are fully informed.

Background Checks

When it comes to background checks, rely on your HR department to provide you with the legal guidance and logistical support. According to Smith & Mazin (2004), "The law requires that the extent of the preemployment background check be appropriate in relation to the specifics of a job." Fortunately, HR professionals are aware of the legal and logistical issues surrounding background checks, so you don't have to worry about that step. If information is uncovered in the background check that would be a disqualifier, you will be notified by HR, as will the the applicant.

A Note About Working with Human Resources

Nurse managers who have mastered the Hiring SMARTT process and have found the right candidate for the right job tend to have something in common: an excellent working relationship with the HR department and the nurse recruiters. Whether the recruiters are part of the nursing department or HR, they are invaluable in the hiring process.

If you haven't done so already, find out the name of your HR liaison for hiring new staff—both nursing staff and ancillary staff. Set up a meeting with your HR partner(s) and start building a relationship by asking questions and listening. There may be more than one person who assists you, so you'll want to meet with each one separately. I asked several nurse recruiters for a list of items they would encourage nurse managers to discuss with their recruiter and compiled the following list:

1. Discuss ground rules for working together. Find out your responsibilities as well as the recruiter's responsibilities.

2. Share your vision of the ideal candidate to fill this position. Be specific about the knowledge, skills, and abilities you are seeking. The nurse recruiters are very interested in this information because it helps them find the best candidate.

3. Ask for a chronological overview of the hiring process. Ask about realistic expectations and timeframes. How often should you check in? How often can you expect to get resumes, information on background checks, etc?

4. Understand the legal side of hiring. Ask for help with writing interview questions. The recruiters I spoke with enjoy sharing their knowledge and expertise; it's there for the taking.

5. Appreciate the challenges the recruiter faces in terms of timing, finding qualified candidates, reference checking, etc. Assume positive intent and try to be patient.

6. Form a relationship of open, direct communication. Take your recruiter to lunch. Send a thank-you note when he or she helps you hire someone marvelous (I put that in—they didn't). This partnership is the key to working well together.

HR can also help you with initial telephone screening, background checks, and reference checks. Generally, your primary responsibility is to interview the candidate, ask the right questions, and seek feedback from others on your team to determine a good fit.

Summary

After the interview, the hiring process is still in full swing. Your ability to review the responses and evaluate the candidates is critical to making the right hiring decision. Keep these elements in mind as you move forward.

- Take good notes so that you have an accurate record of the interview.
- Use a consistent rating scale for all applicants, and make sure other interviewers use the same scale.
- Avoid ingrained biases by checking your beliefs and mindsets in advance of the decision-making process.
- Utilize human resources and the nurse recruiter for prehire testing, references, and background checks.

By carefully reviewing each applicant's responses and evaluating each one, you are ready to make the best hiring decision possible.

CHAPTER 5
Take Your Time Making the Hiring Decision

Hiring SMARTT

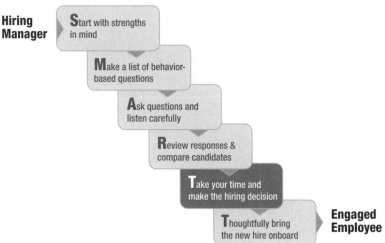

Hiring Manager

Start with strengths in mind

Make a list of behavior-based questions

Ask questions and listen carefully

Review responses & compare candidates

Take your time and make the hiring decision

Thoughtfully bring the new hire onboard

Engaged Employee

It is finally time to make the hiring decision. Is your stomach churning out of fear of hiring someone who will not work out or are you feeling great about the top 2–3 candidates? Either way, the last thing you want is to rush into a decision based on your gut feelings. Many managers (especially those with little experience hiring people) tend to rely on their intuition when hiring and often make up their mind about someone before the candidate has even had a chance to complete the interview. Remember, hiring from the heart is a recipe for disaster.

If you start to feel convinced one way or the other about a candidate early on, slow the process to make sure you are considering all the facts. Listen to your gut, but let your brain inform you, too. Remember, the goal of this process is to find the right fit. You need time, a thoughtful process, and the help of others to achieve this fit. Presumably, an HR representative or a nurse recruiter has been involved in the hiring process up to this point. These folks are a valuable resource when making the decision. The old adage, "two heads are better than one" is definitely true when it comes to Hiring SMARTT.

From One Manager to Another

Bette, a nurse manager at a community teaching hospital said, "You have to know what it is you're looking for. You need to be very clear. Hold true to the vision and culture you are trying to create. Have confidence and stick to your guns. Avoid taking just any 'warm body' at all costs. Patience pays off!"

Of course, no surefire way can guarantee that you select the best candidate. However, you can increase your odds by following this helpful process as you get ready to make the hiring decision.

1. Determine minimum ratings for strengths
2. Chart the ratings for each candidate
3. Get input from others
4. Consider other variables
5. Make a decision based on fit

Love at First Sight

Jamie, a new nurse manager working in pediatrics said, "I knew the instant Gloria walked in the room that she was the person for the job. She radiated positive energy and enthusiasm and that was what we were lacking. We had a great time during the interview, she asked me lots of great questions, and I decided to stop looking and hire her on the spot." Later, I learned that two weeks after Gloria started, Jamie knew that she was wildly enthusiastic and wildly unorganized as well. The nurses who followed her shift (and a few family members) started complaining about her inability to get the work done. Lesson learned: Sometimes "love at first sight" is just infatuation. Take your time and make sure the "marriage" is going to last!

Determining Minimum Ratings for Strengths

Not all strengths are created equal. Some are "nice to have" and others are "need to have." Additionally, the lack of a particular strength can be considered a deal breaker for a candidate. Rob Yeung (2008) calls these hurdles. He says, "The idea for the hurdle rate is to remove quickly candidates who clearly do not meet the requirements for the organization." Remember nature versus nurture; some strengths are teachable and others need to be innate. Hiring someone with the intention of fixing them just does not work. By using a minimum rating score, you weed out the applicants who do not meet your basic requirements.

On a 5-point scale, a proven history of dealing with difficult patients might be more important and therefore have a higher minimum score requirement (hurdle rate) than time management. Both are important, but the first strength might provide a better fit in the department. Additionally, time management strategies can be taught, whereas the ability to deal with difficult people would be a complex topic to convey via training. Review the list of key strengths, and where applicable, create a minimum score that you are seeking.

Charting the Ratings

Comparing the ratings of applicants provides a big picture view of how they measure. A simple way to compare candidates is to create a table, as shown in Table 5.1. In this example, I am using the 5-point scale I recommended in Chapter 4, with 5 being a "Role model" for the strength. (Note that this is a condensed version of the chart. Typically, the left column would include additional strengths.)

Table 5.1   Applicant Comparison Worksheet

	William	Joanne	Martina
Team player	5	4	4
Grace under pressure	4	4	3
Oncology experience Min. Rating = 4	3	4	5
Flexibility Min. Rating = 3	4	3	3
Average	4.0	3.7	3.7

Time-Saver Tools
Applicant Comparison Worksheet   🔲RN

A longer version of this worksheet with boxes to fill in is available for your convenience.

www.HiringFiringInspiring.com

Who do you think is the best candidate based on this rating comparison? You might immediately think William is the man for the job because he received the highest score. Upon closer inspection, William does not meet the minimum requirement for oncology experience. You can assume that the manager selected this minimum score as a result of preceptor resources, past experience, and staffing mix. At this point, Martina seems to be the best choice because Joanne's oncology experience score is lower. This is where the next two steps come into play.

Getting Input from Others

Gathering input from others is wise for two reasons: to avoid personal biases and to create long-term buy-in. You might be thinking, "I don't have biases. I am very objective when it comes to hiring." Well, none of us thinks we show favoritism, but research proves differently. Harvard University researchers have confirmed that we all have subconscious ideas about others that could influence our objectivity. Babcock (2008) says, "Using multiple interviewers with diverse backgrounds and different perspectives is another way to help ensure that more valid and legally defensible selection decisions are made—and that the impact of any biases held by individuals or groups is minimized."

Biases can be as innocent as liking someone because they have children who are similar in age to your children to as prejudicial as disliking someone based on race, age, or gender. Either way, getting others involved in the interviewing and selection process can help you catch any partiality (conscious or otherwise) before it becomes a problem.

When staff members, especially those in informal leadership roles (charge nurses or preceptors), are involved in the interviewing and decision-making process, they are much more likely to support the candidate right from the start. They begin to form a relationship earlier and they have some "skin in the game." The new hire isn't someone you are thrusting upon them; he or she is someone they invited to work in the unit.

Group Decision Making

Maria, a nurse manager on an inpatient psych unit, has an opening for an RN 1. Before the first interview occurs, she wants to make sure that no one is hired who lacks the minimum requirements for the position. She works with two tenured staff nurses, and they decide on the minimum rating for each one. Their focus is finding the candidate who best fits the job as outlined by the list of strengths.

Maria also asks these nurses, and one of the techs, to interview each job candidate. Additionally, she has a charge nurse work with each of the candidates during their share day. Ultimately, she wants input from a variety of sources and seeks buy-in for the hiring decision.

Considering Other Variables

Rating scores and group opinions are very helpful, but sometimes you are still not sure who is the best person to hire. When all things are equal, here are a few other variables to consider. I've included some questions to ask yourself (or the hiring committee) when you are stuck trying to determine which applicant to hire.

- **Enthusiasm**
    - How well did the candidate research the organization and the position?
    - Was he or she positive and encouraging about the job?
    - Are you having to sell the position, or is the applicant genuinely interested?
- **Congruence**
    - Are the applicant's answers to your behavior-based questions consistent?
    - Did the person providing a reference use the same adjectives you would use to describe this person?
    - Was the person's demeanor the same each time that you (or someone else) interacted with him?
- **Logistics**
    - Can the person start working as soon as you need him or her?
    - Will the compensation package meet his or her needs?
    - Are there any "sticking points" (schedule, vacations, sick leave) still outstanding?

Thinking through these key questions can help a candidate rise to the top of the group. This is a prime reason why this step starts with the words "Take your time." Ask the HR staff to assist you with contingency items, such as a drug test, background checks, and references. If an employee "fails" any of these elements, the offer typically is rescinded and you are notified by HR. Don't worry, by following these guidelines, you should have a great second candidate in your selection group, and you can go with Plan B.

Repeat After Me

"If she's a *maybe*, she's a *no*." I heard this advice repeatedly from experienced recruiters and managers. Avoid thinking that somebody is better than nobody. Being stuck with a poor fit will cost you—financially and mentally—in the long run. Repeat after me: *If he's a maybe, he's a no.*

Making the Offer

Finally, you are ready to make the offer. In many health care settings, the HR professional will take care of this for you. Usually, HR also handles salary negotiation, based on years of experience, education, and certification. You and the nurse recruiter should have collaborated throughout the process, so the decision will come as no surprise and he or she will fully support your choice.

The new hire should start when your organization's new employee orientation is offered. Organization-wide orientation is important because new employees need to know the basics of working for your organization before they are ready to dive into the specifics of your department. Typically, items such as vision and values, patient satisfaction, infection control, and compliance are covered in the orientation program that all employees attend when they first start. (I discuss orientation meetings further in Chapter 6.) If your organization does not have a formal orientation process, make sure you (or a qualified preceptor) will be available on the new hire's first day to begin the departmental orientation process. When you make the offer, you should push to have the person start on the first day of formal orientation.

You should let the other applicants you interviewed know that they were not selected. Maintaining a positive relationship with the applicants you did not hire is the right thing to do because you never know what will happen. The candidate may get hired in another department or know other great candidates. Always be courteous and prompt in letting applicants know they have not been selected.

Summary

When taking your time to make the best hiring decision, keep the following points in mind:

1. Rate your candidates and identify your "must haves."
2. Consider other variables besides your ratings from the interview.
3. Use a group of people to avoid hiring "from the heart."

After you make the offer, you still have to make sure your new hire is happy, but the bulk of your work has paid off with your SMARTT hiring practices.

CHAPTER 6
Thoughtfully Bring the New Hire Onboard

Hiring SMARTT

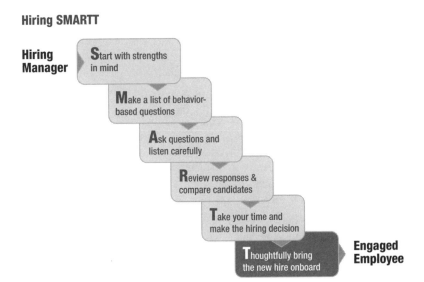

Hiring Manager

Start with strengths in mind

Make a list of behavior-based questions

Ask questions and listen carefully

Review responses & compare candidates

Take your time and make the hiring decision

Thoughtfully bring the new hire onboard

Engaged Employee

You have taken your time to select a candidate who seems to be the right person for the open position. The candidate's strengths meet the organization's needs, the staff supports your decision, and you are starting to breathe a sigh of relief. However, do not be tempted to rest on your laurels just yet. The work of employee engagement starts when the candidate first sees your ad and talks with the HR staff; it continues through your interviews, facilities tour, and share day. Not surprisingly, after the candidate accepts the job, you want to ensure that the new hire feels great about deciding to work in your organization before he or she starts the first day of work.

Staying in Touch

Do you remember the last time you took a new job in a new organization? Remember the feeling of excitement when you said "yes" and received your offer. You let folks in your current job know that you were leaving and everyone wished you well. Starting a new job can be great, but after the initial glow of taking the job fades, doubt often arises. This is why it is important that you, as a manager, stay in touch with a new hire after the offer and before the start date. Staying in touch shows that you care and are invested in the new hire.

Here are a few ideas for staying in touch with a new hire:

- After the candidate accepts the job offer, send a handwritten note welcoming the new hire to your department.

- One week before the new hire's first day, make a phone call stating that you are pleased he or she is starting in a week. Also, ask whether he or she has any questions. Does the new hire know where to park? What to wear? Where to report? Who to ask for?

- The weekend before the new hire starts, send an email reminding him or her of when and where to be on day one. Include your personal phone number (home or cell) so that he or she can call you if necessary.

- Stop by during a break on the first day of orientation. It is easy to say, "HR will handle the orientation from this point," but stopping by to say hello will differentiate you from other managers and make the new hire feel special.

- If the new hire is in orientation for the rest of the week, feel free to set up a lunch meeting later in the week so that he or she can meet the preceptor before coming to the unit.

I suspect that some of you are thinking, "Are you crazy? I do not have time to do all this!" I beg to differ. What would you rather do, invest time now to create a strong foundation or invest time later to deal with engagement issues or to hire the person's replacement? I think most of you will choose to spend time now. Remember, you can also delegate these tasks to other leaders. For example, a charge nurse can write one of the letters or make a phone call.

Let the preceptor take the lead, if that is something that he or she enjoys. Presumably you are not hiring dozens of people, so these initial steps are really a small investment of your time overall.

Lost and All Alone

This story might have an all too familiar ring to it. I think we all know someone who has had a similar experience.

Marcus had completed hospital orientation and nursing orientation. It had been a tough week, but he was anxious to get started on the ortho-neuro unit to which he was assigned. The instructor in nursing orientation said that everyone should report to the unit on Monday morning of the following week. Nervous, Marcus arrived and went to the third floor nurse's station. "I'm here to report for my first day of work." "Huh?" the administrative assistant said. "No one told me you were coming in. Are you sure you're supposed to be here on the third floor?" The charge nurse poked her head into the conversation, "Hey, I'm Alana, can I help you?" Marcus re-introduced himself. "Hmm," she said. "I didn't know you were starting either. Let me call the manager. Who did you talk to?"

Marcus had a rotten feeling in his gut. Had he made the right choice to work on this unit? Maybe his last job hadn't been so bad after all. If this was the first day, could he really expect things to get better? How could his new manager have forgotten he was starting? She had seemed so enthusiastic in the interview. He felt lost and all alone....

You wouldn't want this to happen to you, so don't let it happen to your new hires.

The Department Orientation Process

The new hire is finally ready to begin in your department. Make sure you have everything ready for him or her on the first day of work. If your department requires a specific uniform, ensure the new hire has been fitted and has a uniform. Put his or her picture on the bulletin board and have a locker ready to use. If you have any team-specific welcome items, this is the time to share them. That ICU Nurse coffee mug can be a great surprise on day one!

You want the new hire to feel welcome, and every small detail contributes to showing that you are glad he or she chose to work with you.

If you have not yet done so, now is the time to talk with the nurse educator that works with your unit. In most hospitals, someone in HR or clinical education will assist you with the unit-based orientation process. These folks are trained as educators and are a great resource for partnering with you and your staff to facilitate a smooth orientation. Just as the nurse recruiter was a helpful partner during the hiring process, the nurse or clinical educator is the perfect partner during the onboarding process.

One of our greatest fears in a work setting is looking dumb or unprepared. The last thing a new hire wants to feel is uncomfortable because he or she does not know what to expect. Put your organizational skills to work and provide a thorough orientation process to ease the anxiety level of new hires substantially.

Create an "Orientation Calendar" that includes the following:

- Mandatory organization-wide orientation elements. (In hospitals, this often includes new employee orientation and nursing orientation. In smaller organizations, this might include a meeting with human resources to enroll in benefits and learn about the mission/vision of the organization.)
- Other workshops or certification courses (for example, PALS, ACLS, CPR, etc.)
- Staff meetings
- One-on-one meetings with you
- Work schedule that coincides with the preceptor's schedule (or pre-arranged shifts)
- Field trip or shadow day that is relevant (for example, OR visit)
- Other meetings or events, as appropriate

Time-Saver Tools
Orientation Calendar Guidelines

This fill in the blank calendar with tips and reminders will help you create a thorough orientation calendar for the new hire.

www.HiringFiringInspiring.com

Now, pull out the list of strengths you determined were important for the new hire to possess. Working with the educator and preceptor, create a competency checklist that includes these strengths and others that are necessary in your department for the orientation process. Many organizations have standard checklists that you can access. Use these tools to save yourself a lot of time and energy. One of the primary reasons to have a formal orientation is to validate the skill level of the new person. Hopefully, you have selected an excellent preceptor with whom to share this responsibility.

Picking the Right Preceptor

Great preceptors are special people. At the end of the day, they are role models, counselors, friends, teachers, and much more. Make sure you select the right person for the job (or better yet, let them select the job for themselves).

In an interview with Susan Bindon, MS, RN-BC, senior consultant, education development, for LifeBridge Health, Inc., shared with me the following characteristics an effective preceptor should posses:

- **Interested and willing:** Start by asking for preceptor volunteers. Some organizations ask potential preceptors to complete an application and an interview. A person's willingness is paramount to the long-term success of being a preceptor.

- **Clinically competent:** On the "novice to expert" scale, the goal for a preceptor is mid scale. If a nurse is an "expert," he or she will most likely be *unconsciously competent* (does not have to think about something as he or she does it) and will have forgotten what it takes to do something for the first time. Tapping a preceptor who is consciously competent (thinks about the task while he or she does it) provides a quality connection to the new hire.

- **Realistically patient:** A delicate balance exists between the need to complete assessments and teach new skills and giving the new hire the time and space to perform the new task. Being realistically patient is key.

- **Emotionally intelligent:** An emotionally intelligent preceptor combines self-awareness and social awareness to increase effectiveness when working with others. An effective preceptor has the ability to understand his or her own emotions and empathize with others. Visit the Consortium for Research on Emotional Intelligence in Organizations online at www.eiconsortium.org for excellent information.

- **Able to assess and evaluate competence:** The preceptor must be able to set and write goals to evaluate progress. He or she also must be able to communicate with the orientee about his or her progress toward the desired outcomes. This element encompasses strong assessment skills and assertive communication skills.

- **Good at asking the right questions:** A key part of learning is self-discovery. A good preceptor wants to get the orientee to talk. The process should be more "pull" than "push." When the orientee needs help, an important question is, "What do *you* think you should do now?" (as opposed to simply providing the answer, which is often much easier) followed by, "How did you come up with that set of actions?"

Share the Wealth

Several people I talked with use a co-preceptor model in which two preceptors share the responsibility for orienting the new staff member. This format can help to avoid scheduling conflicts and share the stress of orienting someone. The other benefit (or complication, if handled poorly) is that the new hire has broader support and often learns different ways (all effective, hopefully) to accomplish the same goals. Make sure the preceptors agree on who is responsible for what. You do not want things to fall through the cracks because one person thought the other one was going to handle it. This is a great time to use the nurse educator to help you with the co-preceptor model.

Go to www.vnip.org for more information on preceptors. The Vermont Nurses in Partnership is a nationwide group of nursing professionals whose mission is to "provide educational resources and services that support transitions into the workplace for professional nurses and other staff in health care." The website provides helpful (and free) resources, including preceptor information.

Regular Check-In

Staying in touch with the new hire is a key element of engaging the employee from the start. Even the most experienced new staff member appreciates an opportunity to connect with the hiring manager and talk about how things are going.

Following is a suggested schedule that starts on the employee's first day. For each milestone, where it makes sense, I've included sample questions to ask to elicit feedback. Some of the questions may seem basic, but each one provides you with valuable feedback for engaging this employee. Pay close attention to the responses so that you begin to understand what makes this person tick. This will be very helpful over time in motivating this staff member.

- **During Orientation:**
  — Stop in to say hello at least once (as mentioned earlier) and welcome the new person.
- **Department—Day 1:**
  — Meet and greet the new hire upon arrival.
  — Introduce and hand off to preceptor.
  — If possible, meet with the new hire at end of the first shift. Sample questions:
    • How was your first day?
    • Is there anything I need to help you with before day two?"

- **Department—Week 1:**
  - — Schedule an appointment with the new hire during his or her last shift of week. Sample questions:
    - • How was your first week?
    - • How did this week compare to what you expected?
    - • What resources do you need to feel comfortable moving forward?
    - • How are things working with your preceptor?
- **Department—End of Month 1:**
  - — Schedule a lunch meeting. Sample conversation topics include:
    - • Tell me a little more about yourself (interests; hobbies, etc.)
    - • What's been going well for you this first month?
    - • What's been most challenging?
    - • What suggestions do you have for improving our unit orientation?
    - • If the person fits in and you are happy with the hiring decision and you have other openings in your area, this is a perfect time to ask for the names of former colleagues who might also want to work with you.
    - • Let the new hire know you are happy with his performance and compliment what is going well.

Look Mom, No Hands!

Most of us like to have someone notice when we do something well, especially when we have a new job. We want to prove to others, and ourselves, that we are a contributor. Danielle, a nurse manager for an outpatient surgery center said, "I think of myself as a 'good job' detective when someone is new to the unit. I look for things the person is doing well and compliment him or her regularly. The preceptor is often so focused on areas of improvement that the compliments can fall through the cracks. My recognition of successful interactions with patients, physicians, and colleagues provides the positive reinforcement that I think is critical in the early stages of a job."

90-Day Feedback

I highly recommend that you schedule a formal 90-day feedback meeting with the new hire, the preceptor, and the nurse educator (if applicable). At this point, the orientation checklist should be complete and the new employee should be feeling comfortable on the job. Here are some tips for conducting this meeting:

- Schedule a time when you will not be interrupted and the preceptor and new hire aren't part of the scheduling mix— either before or after a shift.
- Formally thank the preceptor for his or her hard work and assistance during the orientation process by sending a handwritten note, providing a certificate, or some other appropriate form of recognition.
- Review the components of the orientation process, identify any outstanding learning needs, and create an action plan.
- Discuss ways to improve orientation for new hires.
- If applicable, ask the orientee about participating on unit- or organization-wide committees or teams.
- Let the orientee know how he or she will continue to receive formal and informal feedback.
- Before the meeting concludes, ask, "Is there anything else any of you want to talk about?"

I recommend using a checklist like the following to stay on track with each new candidate. Another idea is to put all of the items on your calendar when you hire the new person so that you don't miss important milestones.

Sample Hire to 3-Month Checklist

Date Due	Action Item	Date Completed
	Job offer made and accepted	
Upon acceptance	Handwritten welcome note sent to home address	
1 week before start date	Phone call to check in and answer questions	
Weekend before start date	Email reminder of details for orientation (time, location, dress code, items to bring, etc.) and your phone number	

Time-Saver Tools

Hire to 3-Month Checklist

This expanded version of the checklist includes all of the important components of welcoming a new employee onboard.

www.HiringFiringInspiring.com

Six-Month Check-In

Six months is an exciting milestone for new hires. They should be feeling comfortable at work by now and friendships should be solidifying. They should have a solid comfort level with the work and feel like a positive contributor to the workplace. I talk a lot more in Part II about scheduling a six-month meeting to check in and validate that the employee is a good fit for the job and department.

A performance appraisal form can be a helpful tool for the six-month check-in meeting. Depending on your organization's HR policies, you might complete the form in its entirety or use it as a conversation starter in preparation for the annual review. The new hire should gain a clear understanding of the expectations for his or her performance.

Summary

After you decide to hire a new employee, your journey is not quite over. You need to ensure that the new hire feels welcome and is confident that his or her decision to come to your organization was the correct decision.

1. Send a letter congratulating him or her on becoming part of the staff.
2. Make sure your staff (and preceptor) is ready for the new hire to come to work.
3. Check in with your new employee periodically (1 week, 1 month, 90 days, 6 months) to make sure he or she is happy with the job.

The time you spend initially making your new hire feel welcome should lead to improved engagement, which ultimately leads to better overall performance.

PART II

The Inspiring Manager

At a recent gala celebrating nursing, I heard story after story about how nurses had transformed others' lives, reminding me of how important a nurse's, and by extension, a nurse manager's, role is. As a nurse manager, you have the joy (and sometimes the agony) of being responsible for inspiring not only yourself, but also others. As you know from your clinical training, "inspire" means to "breathe in." When I talk about managers who are inspiring, I am referring to those managers who *breathe life into others*.

A key benefit of inspiring others is the increased employee engagement that inevitably results. Before you can inspire others to be fully engaged, however, you must be inspired and engaged yourself. Making sure you are connected at work is the first step toward inspiring others. Take a few minutes to answer the following questions. Your responses will be very helpful as you move forward.

- What *inspires* you at work?
- What gets you *fully occupied* so time flies?
- When you come to work each morning, what do you *hope to achieve*?

For most people I interviewed, the key element of being inspired at work involves *making a difference*. In your role, you have numerous opportunities to make a difference every day—with your new hire, current staff and co-workers, and of course patients.

Part II focuses on your role as an inspiring manager, for both your new hire and the rest of your staff. I share the key elements of inspiring others using the Partnership Protocol, a guide that I created for busy nurse managers. The Partnership Protocol provides a framework for becoming an inspiring manager. As an inspiring nurse manager, you will notice employees' commitment to their customers and their work improving.

CHAPTER 7
The Partnership Protocol

PARTNERSHIP PROTOCOL™

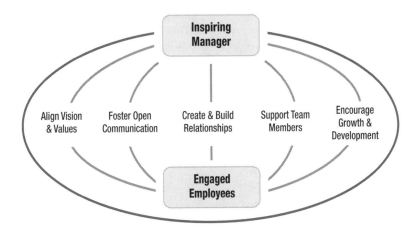

This chapter introduces the Partnership Protocol, an overarching guide for how to be an inspiring manager. The Protocol—a detailed plan that shows that cooperation between you and your staff is the path to long-term employee engagement, positive staff results, and, ultimately, excellent patient outcomes—drives your department's culture. As shown in Figure 7.1, each component of the Protocol starts with a verb to denote an action you take to inspire others. The subsequent chapters of Section II discuss the tools you need to execute the Protocol.

Engaging Employees

At the heart of the Partnership Protocol are engaged employees. The boxes in the model represent action steps that you, as a manager, take to inspire others. Employee engagement is a self-directed endeavor; however, as a manager, you provide avenues and vehicles (either accidentally or on purpose) for employees to become either more or less engaged. Each element of the Partnership Protocol describes one way employees become more engaged through your leadership and inspiration.

Employee engagement is defined in many ways. For the purpose of this book, I am using a definition from Hewitt & Associates, a global human resources consulting firm specializing in employee engagement: "Engagement is the emotional and intellectual commitment of an individual to build and sustain strong business performance" (2009). I chose this definition because it includes an emotional (heart) commitment, an intellectual (head) commitment, and an emphasis on business performance, and I have seen first-hand the importance of all three elements.

Although engagement is a personal matter, as a manager, you can influence your staff both directly and indirectly when you create and maintain a culture of engagement. For example, a direct method of improving engagement is to remove barriers that keep employees from making progress with patients. An indirect method would be demonstrating your own engagement when you act as a positive role model. Many factors create an environment where people can be engaged; being an inspiring manager is only one.

Bigger Fish to Fry

You might be thinking that you have bigger fish to fry than staff engagement. After all, safety, quality of patient care, budgeting concerns, and patient satisfaction are all on your to-do list. Don't be fooled into minimizing the importance of the soft side of health care—the people side.

A study conducted by the Gallup Organization revealed, "Hospitals with higher nurse engagement have statistically lower mortality index and complication index." They go on to say, "Keep in mind that 'engagement' is more than whether employees like their jobs or are satisfied with their manager or benefits. Engagement measures if employees have an emotional bond and psychological commitment to their jobs and their employers" (Paller & Perkins, 2004).

Don't sell yourself short. In your role as an inspiring manager, you have the potential to add significantly to the "emotional bond" and "psychological commitment" parts of the equation. Research shows a positive connection between highly engaged employees, inspiring managers, and better workplace outcomes.

You may be wondering which part of the engagement equation belongs to you and which part belongs to the employee. The Corporate Leadership Council's *Employee Engagement Survey 2004* determined that of the top 25 levels of engagement, 19 were directly connected to the employee's manager. From *clearly articulating goals* to *putting the right people in the right roles at the right times* to *caring about employees*, the study unequivocally shows that a manager plays a major role in engagement.

Because engagement is a personal matter that is influenced by outside conditions, managers need to form a partnership with staff to increase engagement levels and therefore employee performance.

Time-Saver Tools
Partnership Protocol Snapshot Self-Assessment

Wondering how you are doing right now with all the elements of the Partnership Protocol? Take this short assessment as a baseline. Try taking it every six months to see how you progress.

www.HiringFiringInspiring.com

Managing Performance

As the manager of a group of people, you are responsible for making sure that the performance or work that is done by your direct reports is delivered in a manner that is high quality, timely, and helpful. You oversee the team relationships both within and outside your department. You are where the buck stops. Your results as a manager depend on the collective results of the employees who report to you. Because positively impacting your departmental outcomes is the overarching goal of employee engagement, your focus should be on elevating the day-to-day performance of each employee. Because of your commitment to your staff and customers, performance management is a key responsibility of your job.

I define performance management as the process a manager uses to enable employees to do their jobs and to meet the organization's goals. A good part of your day is involved in performance management, whether you realize it or not. All of the following are elements of performance management:

- Sharing organization-wide updates and strategic direction.
- Reviewing goals at a staff meeting.
- Complimenting staff or sharing compliments from others.
- Coaching staff to improve behavior.
- Meeting (formally or informally) to talk about work goals, systems, and processes.
- Conducting formal performance appraisals.

According to talent management experts Development Dimensions International (DDI), "The most effective performance management systems are characterized by their consistent use throughout the organization, their integration with other systems, senior management involvement, employee involvement, and their links to organizational strategy." To make performance management easier to implement day-to-day, I've created an easy way to remember its components: the Performance Platform.

Using the Performance Platform

Sometimes performance management feels like a nebulous term with too many moving parts. As an easy way to remember the basic steps for managing performance, consider the three-legged Performance Platform shown in Figure 7.2.

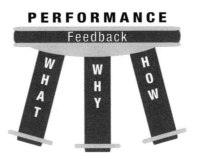

Figure 7.2

The legs elevate performance and represent the *what,* the *why* and the *how* of the desired behaviors. Just under performance lies the feedback you give to staff—both formally and informally. This platform is the foundation for performance management. When you do a good job managing staff performance, retention increases and you will notice fewer involuntary terminations.

What: Sharing Expectations

Performance management starts with letting staff know what you expect from them. During the hiring process, you outline key competencies for the new staff member. Presumably, tenured employees are aware of the key behaviors required for their job. When change occurs and new behaviors are introduced, you need to share what you would like staff members to do differently.

Whether you are delivering new technology, service excellence, or patient care changes, it is important that you clearly state performance expectations. This allows staff to do their best and succeed at work. Without clearly shared expectations, you are just hoping that your staff knows what to do.

When setting expectations, clearly identify what you consider to be good (or great) performance. For example, when describing her hospital's behavioral standards for making a positive first impression, Ashley, a nurse manager focusing on service excellence, includes making eye contact, smiling, introducing yourself, and asking for the person's name. By describing what she wants staff to do, there are no outstanding questions. Everyone knows what Ashley (and the patients) expects.

Why: Sharing Strategic Connection

Hand-in-hand with sharing what behavior you want staff to do is sharing *why* the behavior is important. Staff members appreciate knowing the reason for implementing behavioral change. As a nurse manager, you should share how the desired behaviors connect to the strategic imperatives of your department and organization. For example, Gwen, a nurse manager in the Oncology Department, introduces performance standards to minimize post-surgical nosocomial infections. After explaining what staff members need to do, she connects the procedures to their departmental or organizational goal of decreasing patients' lengths of stay. Employees want to know the *why* as well as the *what;* believe me when I tell you that just saying, "Because I told you so" is not going to cut it.

How: Providing Education and Training

Depending on the complexity of the behaviors, you should provide education and training for employees who are not already competent. This can range from a quick reminder to on-the-job training. For example, while introducing standards for data entry when admitting patients, Christine, a manager in labor and delivery, hands out snapshots of computer screens her staff will see when using the system. She invites someone from nursing informatics to describe the steps for admitting patients to the unit and gives each staff member a small card with shortcuts for entering the information.

Work with your nursing educator or advanced practice nurse (or partner with other nurse managers) to provide necessary education and training to implement expected behavior. If staff members do not know how to implement policies and procedures, your feedback will fall on frustrated ears.

Personalize the Platform

Each person responds to different levels of information when you share the elements of the Performance Platform. An experienced staff member may just need to know the *why* because he or she understands the *what* and the *how.* Someone with less experience may need all three. Get to know your staff and seek to understand what makes them tick. As someone who loves to learn, I enjoy delving into all the nuances of what needs to be done and how to do it. Someone else might want "just the facts" because he or she doesn't care why something needs to be done. Neither of us is right or wrong; our styles of learning and adapting differ. When you use an individualized approach, you find the results are more satisfying and performance improves.

Providing Feedback

The Performance Platform also includes a feedback element. Letting employees know how their performance compares to your expectations is important so that staff know where they stand. Feedback involves complimenting employees when they do a good job and coaching them when they don't. Informal feedback happens on-the-go and is usually short and to the point. Formal feedback occurs in one-on-one meetings, performance appraisals, or the progressive discipline process. I talk more about each of these later in the book.

Feedback Features

Interim Feedback: In Chapter 9, "Foster Open Communications," I discuss the importance of regular one-on-one meetings with each staff member. This is the time to provide interim feedback on performance trends. For example, Dean, a nurse manager in an outpatient surgical center, meets with his direct reports every other month. He keeps a file of compliments for each person and summarizes the trends at each meeting. He reinforces key behaviors and connects them to the desired behaviors that he shared when setting expectations.

Formal Feedback: An annual performance appraisal provides the tool for measuring performance against desired behaviors. Although your organization provides the tool, you make the conversation meaningful to

continues

the employee. For example, Yolanda, a nurse manager in a community health center, schedules one-hour meetings with her staff two times a year for their performance review. During the first meeting, conducted in June, she reviews the goals from the previous year's assessment and discusses progress toward the goals. She asks the employee to talk about his or her goals for the next six months, as well as suggestions to improve the center. This is an informal meeting that lays the groundwork for the formal session, which occurs in December. In the formal meeting, Yolanda reviews each of the sections on the appraisal, shares her rankings, and leaves time for discussion and more goal setting.

Each element of the Performance Platform influences your effectiveness. Your ability to share the *what,* the *why,* and the *how* of performance and your ability to provide feedback on staff execution, greatly affects your role as an inspiring manager.

Time-Saver Tools

Performance Platform Reminder Card

To help you remember the key elements of the Performance Platform, I've created a reminder card for you to print out and put in your pocket or hang on your computer.

www.HiringFiringInspiring.com

Putting the Performance Platform into Practice

Dorothy, an experienced nurse manager in a GI-GU unit, observed that several staff members ignored family members when they approached the nurse's station. Dorothy decided to use the Performance Platform as a guide to improve the behaviors. Because this appeared to be a group problem, she decided to discuss her observations at the next staff meeting. Dorothy figured it had been over a year since the last mandatory workshop on making a great first impression. She took the time to pull out the service behaviors they had all been given to use as a guide at the meeting.

At the staff meeting, Dorothy explained that the unit would be increasing its focus on making excellent first impressions (the *what*). She then talked about patient satisfaction goals and the organization's focus on providing a culture of caring for patients and visitors (the *why*). Finally, she handed out the specific steps for making a great first impression (the *how*).

Over the next few weeks, Dorothy paid close attention to staff members to see how they were doing with the desired behaviors. She provided compliments (informal feedback) when she saw folks doing a great job. She also provided feedback that reiterated the *what,* the *why,* and the *how* of improvement. Additionally, Dorothy shared written compliments and satisfaction surveys from patients that the unit received and provided additional training for staff who still weren't getting it.

After a few months, Dorothy could say with confidence that the department was a role model for excellent first impressions. She celebrated with sweets and treats at a later staff meeting to recognize all the great work the staff had done. The Performance Platform provided the guidance she needed to make the change in the department.

Summary

This chapter introduced the Partnership Protocol, a framework for becoming an inspiring manager. The five elements, discussed in greater detail in subsequent chapters, are as follows:

- Align vision and values.
- Foster open communication.
- Create and build relationships.
- Support team members.
- Encourage growth and development.

Supporting the Partnership Protocol is the Performance Platform, the foundation for elevating employee performance. The elements of the platform are

- What
- Why
- How
- Feedback

Enhanced performance plus solid and steadfast partnerships equals a strong and productive department, with you resolutely at the helm. Ultimately, this combination also results in improved patient-care and business outcomes.

CHAPTER 8
Align Vision and Values

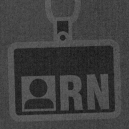

PARTNERSHIP PROTOCOL™

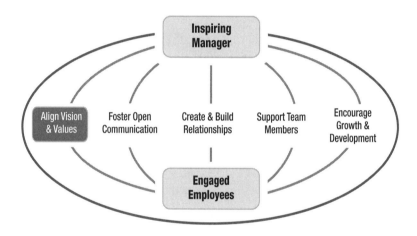

The first section of the Partnership Protocol, introduced in Chapter 7, focuses on aligning the vision and values not because it starts with A, but because this step provides the basis for the other sections. It just makes sense to start with the big picture view so that you and your staff really understand why you do the things you do every day. Here's an example of a vision statement. "Childrens Hospital Los Angeles will be one of the best pediatric medical centers in the world, known for advancing research and providing definitive diagnosis and treatment for our diverse community of children and adolescents with complex diseases" (Childrens Hospital). The vision and values of an organization are the true north, or the guiding ideal, and they are worth talking about on a regular basis. The vision and values help when you are sharing the *why* of the Partnership Protocol's Performance Platform. If the *why* behind the work is missing, the platform will wobble and fall.

Communicating the Vision and Values

Unfortunately, organizational vision and values statements are often thought of as pithy proclamations hung on the walls of hallowed institutions. Do you and the staff know your organization's vision and values? According to the Corporate Leadership Council's *Employee Engagement Survey 2004*, the "most important among the 25 highest-impact drivers of engagement are a connection between employees' job and organizational strategy and employee understanding of how important their job is to organizational success." Since the vision and values drive the organizational strategy, you cannot create this connection if employees don't know the vision and values. Have you found this to be true with you and your staff? How much time do you spend focusing on vision and values versus putting out fires and reacting to everyday struggles in your department?

Unfortunately, I hear many stories from nurses and nurse managers about the difficulties of getting the work done with limited resources. This might lead you to believe that the vision and values can be relegated to the sidelines so that the real work can get done. I disagree. In light of these tough challenges, the roles of the vision and values are more important than ever. The *vision* provides a roadmap for where you are going, and the *values* show you how to get there. Think about planning a vacation with no destination in mind or map to follow. Driving around aimlessly for a little while might be fun, but you would soon tire of either going in circles or accidentally stumbling upon some good place to visit. Having a destination and a map increases your chance of arriving where you want to be. The same idea applies to using the organization's vision and values as an itinerary for your department to move forward.

Using Vision as a Roadmap

Josie, a nurse manager in a rehab unit in a long-term care facility, shared a story of a complaining employee. Henry was dissatisfied with his assignment day after day and came to Josie's office to "vent." Josie is a firm believer in exemplifying the organization's vision, which includes "providing innovative care," as a component of her management style. She also incorporates the values of compassion and quality in her management strategies.

Instead of getting defensive or shrugging off Henry's complaints, she asked Henry, "How can you use the assignment you have been given as an opportunity to provide innovative care to our patients in a high quality and compassionate manner?" Henry did not expect to hear this. He thought Josie would go to the charge nurse and tell her to change his assignment. After some discussion, Henry realized there was an opportunity for him to use some new skills he had learned at an in-service to be more innovative. He thought about how he could be more compassionate in his care and, ultimately, he felt connected to the unit's emphasis on quality. Josie used the vision and values as a roadmap for Henry, and Henry changed his view of the assignment and felt more connected to the unit. Success!

Sometimes, the organization's vision feels too broad. If you feel that way, then adapt a more localized vision that relates to your work area. As a manager, you can examine your organization's or specialty area's vision and focus on the components that apply to your department. Another idea, shared by a nurse manager I interviewed, is to use the vision of a specialty nursing association as a guide. Whatever approach you choose, have a staff meeting to talk about what resonates with your group. Make sure the vision is a living statement, not just a poster on the wall.

Making a Strategic Connection

Making a strategic connection involves sharing with the staff person how his or her job connects to the strategic imperatives of the organization. For example, the nurse understands that his or her response to an individual patient translates to the organization meeting its strategic patient satisfaction goals. Interestingly, in my surveys of nurses and nurse managers, having a strategic connection to the vision and values received a 45% strong influence rating and a 46% moderate influence rating. This was relatively low compared to other areas (such as team support and open communication), which rated much higher levels of influence. Although this challenges the nationwide research done by The Corporate Leadership Council (2004) that I shared earlier, don't throw out the baby with the bath water and totally ignore the vision and values if your opinion is similar to the nurses I interviewed. The bottom line is that more than 90% of respondents said that the strategic connection had some level of influence, so pay attention to the vision and values.

If you have never focused on creating a strategic connection and sharing the vision and values with others, now is a good time to try. If you do not already have them, ask your boss for a copy of the organization's strategic initiatives. Have a discussion with your manager to clearly identify the connection in your area of work. Then share the strategic initiatives and make the connection to the vision and values. Nurses working in organizations that are trying to achieve Magnet status report feeling a positive connection to a bigger goal—a vision for their practice.

Another part of creating a strategic connection is shared values. Shared values are the way in which work gets done. Values such as patient-centered care, respect, and teamwork give staff direction on how work should be done. You can use shared values as a gauge for quality patient care when you talk about desired outcomes and use the values in your discussions.

Remember that values are the way you get to the destination. Feel free to discuss how to maintain the pledge to the values despite high stress and difficult situations. Values are foundational because they serve as a guide, especially when staff members are under pressure. At the very least, you want to pick a lane when it comes to vision and values. Wavering back and forth and putting out conflicting messages is like driving under the influence of inconsistency and a lack of direction.

Establishing a Department Brand

You have an internal brand in your department whether you think you do or not. For our purposes, your brand is what people think about your department—an identity of sorts that others relate to your area. When I worked on a postpartum unit, I would describe the brand as high touch; high quality of care. We had a broad array of patients, from highly educated and demanding to drug addicted and underserved mothers and their babies. Our brand (and the organization's vision) revolved around providing equally high quality care for all.

Think of the places where you have worked. How would you describe the brand of that department or others you observed? Your department might value a sense of calmness, of being laid back, whereas another department might be known for its commitment to learning and development. Others might pride themselves on a sense of teamwork and partnership or research and cutting-edge innovations.

Here's an exercise to determine your department's brand. Finish these sentences and then ask five (or more) staff members to finish them as well.

- Our department is best known for…
- When you come into our department, you feel…
- For someone to "fit" on our unit, he or she must be…
- We take pride that our department consistently…
- Something that will never change here is…

These may look familiar because they also relate to finding the right fit from the earlier Hiring section. You also want the staff to feel the fit day-in and day-out. Building a brand will help you accomplish this goal.

Time-Saver Tools

Department Brand Exercise

I've put the questions listed earlier in an exercise you can use with staff members to clearly define your department brand. Remember to have fun when you do this.

www.HiringFiringInspiring.com

Step Outside the Box

The marketing department in your organization most likely works hard to create an external brand for your organization—the brand they want the public to relate to. These people are a great resource for creating and implementing an internal brand for your area. Find out the name of a peer in the marketing department. Call and invite him or her to lunch. Brainstorm together about how to tie your internal brand to the external messaging that employees hear in the media. LifeBridge Health, Inc. (www.LifeBridgeHealth.org), a large health system in Baltimore, Maryland, has a marketing campaign that revolves around the slogan, "The Freedom to…" The campaign includes stories of staff members exercising their "Freedom to Excel," "Freedom to Sing," "Freedom to Learn," and so on. As a nurse manager, you could use this messaging as a way to communicate your desire for staff to share the "Freedom to… (fill in the blank)."

After clearly identifying the brand, have fun sharing the message. Here are a few ideas to get started. Suppose that your brand is "Professional Paradise" and your vision is "Satisfied, energized, and productive staff who provide high-quality patient care."

- Include the brand in your staff meeting announcements, agenda, minutes, reports, and so on.
- Title your newsletter so that it relates to your brand—for example, *Postcards from Professional Paradise.*

- Add some tropical clip art to the fliers you post around your unit to convey your internal brand.

- Hang tropical decorations in the break room or locker room.

- Bring Caribbean food to your next department potluck lunch. Find out about random holidays that are related (Hawaii Day?).

You get the idea.

Being a Positive Role Model

If you want staff members to align their actions with the vision and values of your organization, you must be a positive role model. As a nurse manager, *you* are a key element of your brand. In a survey I conducted with nurses, a common theme was the desire for the nurse manager to be a strong role model. Comments included "being the calm in the storm" or "having a sense of humor." Additionally, when I conducted focus groups with nurse managers, a common theme was being a positive role model. One nurse manager said, "I am a mirror for my unit." She went on to say that she wants emotions to be in check on the unit, so she has to keep her emotions in check. Some nurse managers reported taking on the role of a parent. If you are feeling like a parent in your department, then the staff might be feeling like children. That's not good for anyone.

A key element of being a positive role model is to maintain your poise in challenging situations. When you reach a stumbling block, try to turn it into a stepping-stone by using the SHIFT™ technique. SHIFT is an acronym. The process includes five steps for handling tough situations and people. As a manager, you will not always be able to control which obstacles come your way, but you can always control your response to these challenges. Using these steps helps you in your quest to be a positive role model.

SHIFT Steps

Stop and breathe.

Harness harmful, knee-jerk reactions.

Identify and manage negative emotions.

Find new options.

Take one positive action.

Let's dive in and look at each step. Imagine that you've just experienced a stressful situation at work. Now…

Stop and Breathe

Notice that you are feeling stress or anger? If you are alone in your office or car, speak the word, "Stop!" If you are in a crowd, say it in your head. Then take a deep cleansing breath. This step gives you the time you need to collect yourself.

Harness Harmful, Knee-Jerk Reactions

Knee-jerk reactions are automatic, unthinking responses. They can range from storming out of a room to becoming a shrinking violet and anything in between—raising your voice, complaining, sulking, talking fast, name calling, blaming others, and talking about people behind their back. In a negative situation, harmful reactions usually fall into the fight or flight category, and are often unproductive. Everyone benefits when you harness your negative knee-jerk reactions, but you benefit the most.

Identify and Manage Negative Emotions

Stressful situations usually create negative emotions. Negative emotions, left unchecked, can cause trouble in any number of work situations. Therefore, the **I** in SHIFT represents identifying the negative emotions you're experiencing. You must make a conscious effort to notice that you feel these emotions and then name them. The second part of this step is to manage the emotions. Once you know which emotions you're dealing with, you can choose to break the pattern. This step is about learning how to flip the switch (in a helpful way) on your emotions in order to remain calm.

Find New Options

Take a few minutes to consider (find) new options that move you closer to less stress and positive results. Reflect on what you have done in the past that worked well in a similar situation; you also might think of how someone you admire would handle things. These steps put you in a more proactive position instead of a reactive one.

Align your options with the vision and values of the department and organization when responding to tough situations and finding new options. Consciously creating choices provides a feeling of being in control that most people appreciate and lessens your stress in the long run. Being creative and thinking of a variety of options opens up possibilities that may have gone unnoticed in the past.

Take One Positive Action

After you discover new possibilities, the final step is to choose at least one that feels right for the situation and take action! Take what was merely positive thinking and move it toward reality. Remember thoughts alone rarely achieve anything. You must *act* if you want a better outcome.

That's it. The SHIFT steps can revolutionize your ability to get to and stay in Professional Paradise. Want help remembering the steps or examples of other ways to use the SHIFT process? Visit www.ProfessionalParadise.com to download the free tools.

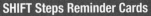

Time-Saver Tools
SHIFT Steps Reminder Cards

Once you've mastered the SHIFT steps, you can teach it to others. Feel free to print out these reminder cards to give to staff as an easy way to remember.

www.HiringFiringInspiring.com

Summary

Aligning the vision and values of the organization with the roles and expectations of the staff is a key responsibility of the nurse manager. Without proper direction and a guide for getting there, your staff will feel less connected to the higher purpose of health care. Your belief and support of the department's vision and values gives you a foundation from which to lead. The way you demonstrate your vision and values is translated to an internal brand, which allows new and experienced staff to work from this foundation as well.

When it comes to aligning vision and values, your ability to be a role model is key. Your direct reports want to see your positive attitude, your ability to remain calm in the storm, and your sense of humor. You become a living example of the vision and values for all to see.

CHAPTER 9
Foster Open Communication

PARTNERSHIP PROTOCOL™

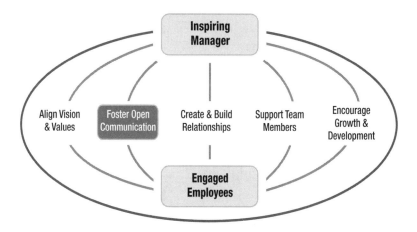

As a nurse manager, you are communicating from the moment you arrive at your workplace. Even if you do not say a word, your staff is already figuring out whether this will be a good day or a bad day based on your body language. The overwhelming evidence from surveys and focus groups I conducted and from research from other sources is that communication is a key element of inspiring (or de-motivating) employees and forming a strong partnership with staff. Communication skills, from positive reinforcement to having uncomfortable conversations regarding performance, play a vital role in engaging employees.

When nurses are asked, "What should your nurse manager continue to do," the majority of responses include comments related to open, honest, consistent communication. From open-door policies and hallway huddles to one-on-one meetings and performance reviews, inspiring nurse managers use communication to engage with employees.

We learned as youngsters that it's not what you say but how you say it, so it should be no surprise that nurses want their managers to communicate in positive ways. Whether you are communicating formally or informally, your role as a manager includes many aspects of verbal, non-verbal, and written communication. The following sections focus on those areas that are relevant to nurse managers, as reported to me in research, survey findings, and focus group settings:

- Communication style
- Communication methods
- Coaching communication

Communication Style

At its most basic level, the communication process involves a sender, a message, a channel, and a receiver (Leaf, 2005). As a manager, you should pay special attention to all four elements to ensure that your message is conveyed effectively. Your style, the way you choose to communicate, ultimately has a direct connection to your relationship (or lack thereof) with your staff. There is no perfect communication style. However, the words I heard repeatedly were "be consistent" and "be fair."

Your communication style is influenced by your personality, past experiences, and formal learning. You demonstrate your style through your words, tone, and body language. Dr. Albert Mehrabian, professor emeritus of psychology, University of California, Los Angeles, conducted research that confirms that when it comes to likeability, your words account for 7% of your message, tone of voice accounts for 38%, and body language accounts for 55% (Johnson, 2007). "Likeability" is what Mehrabian measured in his study, but his research has held the test of time and the statistics transfer to other elements of communication besides likeability. The point here is that your ability to communicate is more about how you say something than what you say.

So what's a busy manager to do? Start by using the SHIFT steps discussed in Chapter 8. If there is any chance that your body language or tone can be misconstrued as a knee-jerk reaction or negative emotion, take a moment to pull back and get yourself together (unless, of course, you *want* someone to see your frustration, anger, or disappointment). Over time, your staff will count on your ability to stay calm in the storm. Your ability to manage your response to others is a key factor of building positive relationships with members of your staff.

Sometimes, managers think they are communicating well, but others disagree. We all have blind spots—barriers to communication that we raise and that others see, but we don't. Blind spots are the equivalent of having spinach in your teeth or paper on your shoe. You think you look good, but others know better. To uncover your communication blind spots, here are some questions to ask a trusted peer or direct report, or your boss:

- I am working on improving my communication skills, what should I stop doing?
- What should I continue doing?
- What should I start doing?

You have to be willing to listen. Feel free to take notes, but no commenting on the comments. You can ask follow-up questions if the feedback is unclear, but this is not the time to disagree with or challenge the person. Just say, "Thank you."

YAY! She's Gone

A group of nurses that work the evening shift on a post surgical unit shared a story about their manager, Naomi. "Naomi isn't very good at hiding her feelings," reported one of the nurses. "We always know when something is on her mind. I know she tries to act like everything is okay, but we can tell when it isn't," added a second nurse. "She needs to get control of her emotions. When she acts stressed, it's contagious, and not in a good way. The best part of our shift is when Naomi goes home. We can all breathe easier and get back to our work."

No manager wants the staff to be happy when he or she leaves. The prescription for Naomi is to discover her blind spots. She needs to ask for and listen to feedback. Then, of course, get help to change her communication methods—verbal and non-verbal—and then ask for feedback again. Naomi's goal should be to hear, "Yay! Naomi's here!"

Communication Methods

This section discusses the following methods of communication for nurse managers:

- Informal communication
- One-on-one communication
- Group communication
- Electronic communication

Informal Communication

Informal communication occurs during those times when you are talking with a member of your staff on-the-fly. When you are in your department, if you see someone doing a good job and you comment on it, you are engaging in informal communication. Another example would be poking your head in on the shift report to ask how things are going, You have no formulated plan for what you are going to say; you just make the effort to be with staff in a more relaxed setting.

Without informal communication, your staff may feel disconnected from you, wonder what you are thinking, or question whether something is going on. The trick is finding the balance between seeing how things are going and micromanaging. When you arrive on the unit and pick out things that are wrong or jump in and take over without asking, you give the impression that you don't trust the staff and this can damage your partnership with them.

The overriding goal of informal communication is to stay in touch and let folks know that you care about what's happening. Additionally, if you are communicating informally on a regular basis, coming around to make a suggestion becomes no big deal.

Consistency Counts

D. Morrison, RN, BSN, MBA, OCN, and newly hired nurse manager at Sinai Hospital of Baltimore, Maryland, shares this sage advice with her peers (personal communication, December 2, 2009.). "I find that consistency [in communication] works. As a new manager, staff will sometimes 'test' you. Different people will ask the same questions in a different way in an effort to get to you agree to something outside of standard procedure. An example would be: Staff is not allowed vacation between December 15th and January 15th. Two people have asked in some form or another if they can just have one day or more because family is visiting or they are traveling out of town. This is not a new policy, but it appears since I'm new here, maybe I don't know or would just say 'okay.'"

Stick to your guns and show consistency in your communication so that staff members understand your commitment to the department.

One-on-One Communication

One-on-one meetings can lead to a rich partnership with staff members. Keep communication open, honest, and consistent, and staff will see over time that you are trustworthy. When you take the time to listen thoughtfully, bounce around ideas to solve problems, and inject your sense of humor into every day challenges, your relationship becomes more comfortable and more productive. In my national nurse survey, 86% of nurses said that creating an environment of trust within the unit or department had a strong influence on their commitment, performance, and work effort.

The one-on-one meeting is a great time to provide formal feedback from the Performance Platform (refer to Chapter 7). You can also find out if staff members who are not reaching their potential are missing the *what,* the *why,* or the *how* by asking questions and listening carefully. One nurse manager wrote on her survey, "One-on-one discussions have been great in gaining insight into the changes we have made for the unit and for staff buy-in." Although often reluctant to admit it, most employees enjoy one-on-one meetings with their supervisor.

The One-on-One Meeting Agenda

Many nurse managers fear that holding regular one-on-one meetings will take too much time. To make the system easier and less time-consuming, use a standard agenda. When you sit down to prepare for the meeting, you will have a built-in set of questions as a guide for what to discuss.

The agenda for a one-on-one meeting can be fluid and flexible.

1. **What works?** Start with the good news. Ask the direct report to share things that have been going well; then, you share your thoughts on the same subject.

2. **What needs work?** Ask for ideas and suggestions for improving the department. Make sure that the meeting does not turn into a gripe session by challenging the employee to propose solutions.

3. **What's next?** Summarize any action items discussed and agree on who is responsible, the time frame, and the method of accountability.

Be aware of employees who try to get monkeys off their back and pass them to you. Share the responsibility for problem solving; do not take ownership of all the problems. Ask the person, "What do you think you could do to fix that?" instead of saying, "I'll take care of it." One goal of regular communication is employees having the tools (and permission) to act like an owner and take on informal leadership roles while being highly engaged at work.

One-on-one meetings are also great when big changes are occurring in your area, such as new leadership, new technology, or a change in the mix of patients. If you are a new nurse manager, conducting one-on-one meetings is pivotal in creating a strong partnership with your staff, which leads to higher employee engagement and ultimately better results in your department. A new nurse manager in an IV therapy department said, "The first thing I did was meet with each of the staff members individually to explain my role and to listen to what they felt were the problems within the department and ways I could help to improve their work load. This proved to be very effective. They were able to give me some valuable input, and the department eventually ran very smoothly and they had structure, which had been lacking in the past."

Loose Lips Sink Ships

Confidentiality is a critical element of building and maintaining trust. What happens in the one-on-one stays in the one-on-one (unless both parties agree to share information with others). Jan, a staff nurse on a burn unit, shared, "My manager, Riley, loved to talk about my co-workers to me. I kept wondering whether he was talking about me to them. From then on, I watched what I said to him." Can you blame her? Remember, discretion is the better part of valor.

Time-Saver Tools
One-on-One Meeting Template

To save you time, this template provides the agenda for your one-on-one meeting and space to take notes to keep in the employee's file.
www.HiringFiringInspiring.com

Group Communication

Sometimes you want to get information to a group of staff at the same time. You either want to save time or make sure the information is consistent (or both). Group communication is one method to accomplish these goals. Staff meetings are the main example of this type of group communication.

When done well, staff meetings provide a setting for effective communication. Staff meetings should be a dialogue, not a diatribe. Allowing for two-way communication gives staff members a chance to have their voices heard. Nurses also want to be informed about what is happening in the department and organization. They report that they enjoy hearing what is happening outside of their area so they have a context in which to work that connects them to the vision and values of the organization.

Nurse managers sometimes fall into the "no news is good news" trap at meetings. You have known about something for so long that you assume that others know it, too. Or, you have had time to adjust to the news, but the staff has not. Disseminate the necessary information, be patient, and give folks a chance to process what you share. Even when people are open to change, the process is not always easy.

You should schedule meetings to allow optimum attendance across shifts. Many managers ask for staff input before the meeting. Using updated technology, such as teleconferencing, allows people who cannot attend physically to hear the message as well.

As a last resort, recording and sharing minutes helps keep people in the loop if they miss the meeting.

Here's a sample agenda for a staff meeting; of course, you'll want to add your own flair to keep things interesting.

1. **Reconnect with the vision and values (your internal brand):** A great way to dialogue about shared values and responsibilities is to recognize individual staff members or team efforts. Ask others to share good news, too, and then relate it to the vision and values as well.

2. **Share updates:** Share news from management meetings, including strategic initiatives, budget information, reimbursement for services rendered, and so on. When asked, "What should your nurse manager continue to do?" one nurse responded, "Communicating. Our institution is going through some trying times, and she tries very hard to dispel rumors and update the department on new information." Your direct reports will appreciate your candor and openness when it comes to keeping them informed.

3. **Take suggestions:** Open the floor for staff to share their suggestions. Be clear that the topic is not "problems to solve" but "suggestions for improvement." You can use traditional brainstorming techniques, small group discussions, or a pros and cons list to help determine any next steps.

4. **Gratitude and wrap up:** Invite staff to share what they are grateful for. This allows for some positive reinforcement and public appreciation before leaving on a good note.

Time-Saver Tools
Staff Meeting Agenda

You guessed it. To save you time and energy, I've created a staff meeting template including the agenda items outlined earlier. You can include notes on this and use it for communicating the minutes of the meeting as well.

www.HiringFiringInspiring.com

Electronic Communication

The last method of communication is electronic communication—namely e-mail. Remember the Mehrabian statistics I shared earlier that said that 7% of communication is words and 93% is your tone and body language (Johnson, 2007)? Although this research was conducted before e-mail existed, the statistics stand up when applied to electronic communication. Beebe & Masterson (2003) have found that loss of nonverbal cues is one of the foremost concerns when using electronic communication. That's logical; think of e-mails you've received where you thought the sender meant one thing and after digging deeper you found the sender's intent was entirely different.

Use e-mail for sharing statistics, facts, dates, and "non-emotional" data. E-mail is never a good choice for coaching or performance management because you will be missing the non-verbal components of the communication process which clarify the true intent of your words. I can say "great job" with a sarcastic tone and it has a completely different meaning than if I sound genuine and sincere. In electronic communcation, the intended meaning may not always be clear. Sometimes a passive or passive-aggressive response is to shoot off an e-mail to avoid a face-to-face dialogue about a disagreement. This will only lead to trouble in the long run.

E-mail Rules of Thumb

To ensure that your e-mail is most effective, follow these rules :

- Use a relevant subject line—if the subject of the e-mail chain has changed—change the subject line to reflect that update.
- Start with an appropriate greeting—it doesn't take that long to begin with "good morning" or something similar.
- Keep the message short and sweet—if you're working on the second page, you should probably create a more permanent document and attach the file.
- Articulate next steps at the end of the e-mail and who is responsible.
- Answer all e-mails—even if it's just to say, "Got it" or "I'll get back to you." Don't leave people wondering if you are there or not.
- Include an e-mail signature with all your contact information.

- Copy only the people who are relevant to the conversation. You do not want to be that person who is always covering your bases and causing e-mail "pollution."
- Only forward e-mails to those who need the information.

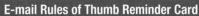

Time-Saver Tools

E-mail Rules of Thumb Reminder Card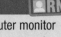

Print out this reminder card and post it on your computer monitor to keep the elements of effective e-mails where they are easy to see.

www.HiringFiringInspiring.com

Coaching Communication

In Chapter 7, I defined performance management as the process a manager uses to enable employees to do their jobs to meet the organization's goals. One key element of performance management is coaching staff to improve behavior. The Performance Platform was introduced as a tool for understanding the basic steps of managing performance. In this section on coaching communication, I will share more specific ideas for how you as a manager can coach employees via your day-to-day conversations.

Coaching communication focuses on improving employee performance to meet the organization's goals and objectives. This coaching can be related to performance that needs to be changed or to performance that you would like to see repeated. Make sure you spend time focusing on both.

One reason this is so important is that a lack of consistent coaching, which is evident in many work environments, causes problems. A theme within the nurses' responses to how nurse managers could be more effective was the need for consistent coaching of staff. Three quotes from the national survey I conducted reflect the frustration of nurses. "I wish my nurse manager would stop ignoring the disruptive behavior of staff members who simply refuse to do what is outlined in their job descriptions." "Stop showing favoritism." "Stop keeping low performing employees." As managers, sometimes we mistakenly think that coaching communication can damage relationships, whereas my experience clearly indicates that it can help to foster open communication and build trust in the long run.

When coaching employees, use the Performance Platform as your guide. After you have communicated the *what,* the *why*, and the *how* to the staff member, provide informal feedback on how the person is doing. Give yourself time to think about what you will say, when you will say it, and the ultimate outcome you seek. I focus on progressive discipline in Part III of the book. For now, the focus is on the *what* and the *how* of coaching.

Many times, managers focus almost exclusively on the improvement side of coaching and forget to recognize a job well done. You are so busy that you forget to compliment folks. People love to get compliments, but only if they are warranted and sincere. When asked, "What should your nurse manager start doing?" survey respondents replied:

- Provide feedback more often.
- Give positive feedback.
- Be positive and affirming.
- Give more praise.

Sticky Note System

B. Bartels (personal communication, 2009), senior HR business partner at St. Joseph Medical Center, shared this great idea for nurse managers. Put a small pad of sticky notes in your left hand pocket every morning. As you walk around and notice staff doing things well, or talk with staff about areas that need improvement, jot down the date, name, behavior, and what you did about it. Now move the sticky note to your right pocket.

At the end of each day, put the notes in a file that you have for each staff member. When you are ready for evaluation time or a one-on-one meeting, you have a helpful record of trends that you noticed. In the world of HR and management, if it isn't written down, it didn't happen.

> April 25, Tiffany
> helped family member
> connect with social
> worker for discharge
> of patient despite
> being busy. Smiled;
> very thorough. I
> complimented her at
> the nurse's station.

When you recognize positive behaviors, remember to make compliments timely, sincere, consistently delivered, meaningful, and personal. "Good job" or "Great day everybody" does not meet this criteria. Employees don't want a superficial pat on the back; they want you to notice what they've done well and comment on it to them personally.

Here's an example of a compliment that meets the criteria above. "I heard it took quite a bit of work yesterday to find the missing information for the chart. Thanks for being so thorough and making us all look good. That's a great example of teamwork for our department! Keep up the great work." A compliment such as this takes a few more seconds, but the impact is much more powerful. Take the time to offer sincere, well-thought-out compliments (and note them in the employee's folder) and everyone benefits.

Is Your Head in the Sand?

When a performance issue comes to the manager's attention, some choices for moving forward are more productive than others. You can

- Look the other way and hope the behavior changes.
- Make a joke with the employee.
- Jot down a note and see if there's a trend.
- Complain to someone else.
- Address the issue.

continues

Unfortunately, many managers choose a passive approach and shy away from coaching because they are afraid it will damage relationships with staff. Down deep, they worry that the staff might not like them. If your coaching style is fair and consistent, your staff may not like what you are saying, but they will respect you for saying it.

When employees are not performing to your expectations, look at where the deficit is coming from. Performance involves three elements.

- **Ability:** If the problem is related to a lack of ability, offer resources and training to improve the skill.
- **Opportunity:** If a lack of opportunity is causing the performance gap, create written procedures that are easy to follow for the few times staff must complete this task.
- **Motivation:** Many coaching opportunities stem from a lack of motivation and this is the most challenging gap to correct. Motivation is internal and is the result of many factors.

Regardless of the cause of the performance gap, you start coaching by clearly sharing your expectations with staff—by sharing the *what, how,* and *why* of the performance. This step was described in Chapter 7 using the Performance Platform. If you haven't communicated the desired outcomes and you start coaching, then staff members have every right to be frustrated. You are giving them feedback on something that they may not be clear on in the first place. Remember, the Performance Platform has three legs—all of which are important to elevating performance. If the *what,* the *why,* or the *how* is missing, the platform will be shaky at best.

The Telephone Game

Remember the telephone game you played as a child, in which one person whispered a message to the next and it was passed along until the last person said the message out loud? Everyone ended up in a fit of giggles because the message was always different from the original words. Unfortunately, some nurse managers use this method of communication—expecting employees to pass along information from one to another—to share information.

Kathleen, a nurse manager in a large clinic, announced a new policy regarding signing in patients. She explained it to members of the morning shift and asked them to share the information with other staff as they arrived. As you can imagine, this "telephone game" version of communication did not work and the evening shift heard bits and pieces of the policy. When Kathleen showed up a few days later during the late hours and started offering coaching suggestions, the staff members were upset because they had never been properly trained on the new policy. Kathleen failed to share the *what,* the *why,* or the *how* with all staff members, and her feedback was not well received. Make sure you communicate desired outcomes to everyone involved before you start coaching.

To address performance issues, especially those that stem from unmotivated employees, I created the DATA Driven Discussion™ model. As the name implies, this model focuses on data and minimizes the focus on emotion. In your coaching, if you focus on subjective information (how people feel) versus objective information (what happened), you run the risk of the coaching turning into a full-blown argument. Fortunately, the DATA Driven Discussion model minimizes the chance of this happening.

Here are four simple steps for conducting a coaching conversation.

- **D**escribe the situation.
- **A**sk questions and listen.
- **T**alk through solutions.
- **A**gree on next steps.

Because patient satisfaction is a desired outcome in every aspect of healthcare and an area where unmotivated staff can have a significant negative impact, I will share how a DATA-driven discussion might sound after a patient complaint. Robert is the manager, and Emily is the nursing tech.

Robert: "Emily, I need to talk with you about something. Let's go in this alcove so we have some privacy. While I was rounding, Mr. Watkins's family said that he hadn't been bathed in two days. I see you took care of him yesterday and today. What's happening with his baths?"

Emily: "Every time I try to bathe him, the family is there, and they ask me to come back later. When they finally left, I was tied up with a new admission. They are so annoying and always in the way. Besides, we were short staffed yesterday because Juanita called in sick. You should be having this conversation with her."

Robert: "It sounds like a couple of different circumstances got in the way of the bath. You know from our protocols that patients need to be bathed every day. What ideas do you have for making sure this happens regardless of the family and staffing?"

Emily: "I don't know. You're the manager. What do you think?"

Robert: "I know you are usually very good at getting baths in—even on busy days. What have you done in the past that worked well?"

Emily: "A few times, I have teamed up with another tech, and we've done them together. Another time I just had to ask the family to leave when I was available, and that worked out okay. I'm just frustrated because it seems like every time someone calls in sick, I get the brunt of the work."

Robert: "I hear your frustration. I think both of your ideas will work in the future. Do we agree that you will bathe the patients every day from now on and that you will go and bathe Mr. Watkins now? I'll work on the staffing side of things and you can always let the charge nurse or me know if you are swamped so we can work with you to get everything done. Thanks for your help with this. I'll follow up with the family."

Notice how Robert was not wrapped up in the emotion that Emily brought to the conversation. He maintained the focus on her performance (or lack thereof). The DATA Driven Discussion model provides you with a roadmap for coaching conversations and over time, employees are more likely to appreciate your feedback because you are consistent and fair.

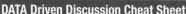

Time-Saver Tools

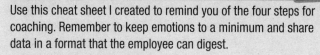

DATA Driven Discussion Cheat Sheet

Use this cheat sheet I created to remind you of the four steps for coaching. Remember to keep emotions to a minimum and share data in a format that the employee can digest.

www.HiringFiringInspiring.com

No Surprises

The annual performance appraisal is a written confirmation of coaching conversations that have happened throughout the course of the year. Anything you write down should have already been discussed, either formally or informally. Remember that folder that I suggested you create to drop notes into to keep up with the employee's progress? Use it as your guide for ranking the employee against the organizational standards. Make sure you have a steady flow of communication around performance so that the annual review is just formal documentation of what's already been said. Remember, no surprises!

Summary

Nurses want a manager who uses a consistent, fair style of communication. Open communication paves the way for building solid relationships and supporting team members. At the end of the day, employees know whether they've done a good job. If you ignore their poor performance, they will continue with bad behavior. If you ignore their good performance, they might slip into unproductive habits. Uncover blind spots in your overall style. Then, employ both formal and informal methods of communication. Finally, offer consistent coaching so that staff members know what you expect and can meet those expectations.

CHAPTER 10
Create and Build Relationships

PARTNERSHIP PROTOCOL™

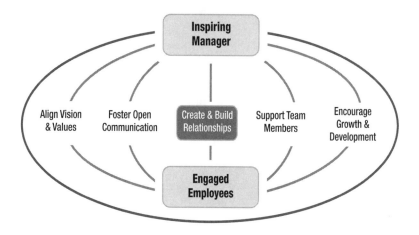

Strong and trusting relationships, which result from the alignment of the vision and values and which foster open communication, play a major role in your ability to get your job done. After all, you cannot possibly complete every task on your own; hence, the Partnership Protocol concept. Creating and building relationships is a critical component of the Partnership Protocol and is vital to inspiring your staff.

Blessing White, a global consulting firm dedicated to creating sustainable high-performance organizations, in their *Employee Engagement Report* (2005), found that "the manager-employee relationship represents a crucial ingredient in the employee engagement formula...good manager-employee relationships smooth the way for mutually beneficial connections between individual employees and their employer." This and other research shows that these mutually beneficial connections lead to better performance, higher staff retention rates, and stronger business outcomes.

To create and build strong relationships, you want to focus on four main areas:

- Maintaining an open-door policy
- Spending time with staff
- Encouraging autonomy
- Keeping a professional distance

Each of these focus areas has at its core an element of trust. When staff members trust you, they are more likely to do a better job, stay longer, and give work their all. At its most basic level, trust is doing what you say you will do. Employees who report to you need to know that you are consistent and reliable in your words and deeds. Don't worry if you're not the touchy-feely type. You don't have to hold hands and sing *Kumbaya*. Just start by becoming more intentional about growing the relationships with staff, and then you can watch workplace results improve as those relationships strengthen.

Maintaining an Open-Door Policy

Having an open-door policy (literally and metaphorically) is a great way for direct reports to informally communicate with you. (Of course, formal communication has established channels already, so the informal communication really is what you will foster with an open-door policy.) An open-door policy simply means that you and your office are open to anyone who wants your time and attention (within reason). Your willingness to let people drop in and talk will prove helpful for at least a couple of reasons: You get to hear about what is working and not working with employees, and you can provide a "safe" place for them to complain. Creating this safe place helps to build trust with employees. In focus groups I lead, experienced nurse managers repeatedly share the value of an open door for nurturing positive relationships.

Depending on where your office is located, you might need to set up a space within the department where staff can find you. Unfortunately, in many facilities, when nurse managers oversee several units, the office may be some distance from the work area. If this is the case for you, be sure you are rounding in your areas daily so that folks can talk with you if they want to. This is the equivalent of carrying your open door around with you. If you are in your department, attempt to find an out-of-the-way place to talk to respect confidentiality. The point of the open door is that you are accessible and employees have your attention. Employees want to know that you are an open and trusted person to talk with and that your office is a safe place.

The Las Vegas Phenomenon

Matthew, a nurse manager in a small community hospital, thinks of his office as Las Vegas for the staff. He says, "They know they can come in here to vent if they are frustrated, they can rant and rave, and I'll just listen. What happens in my office stays in my office." He laughed and said, "My staff know that I won't try to solve the problem or get too involved." After they finish venting, he says he might ask a few questions if he thinks some follow up is needed. Otherwise, he asks whether they need anything else from him, and usually the answer is "No thanks—I just needed a place to vent."

The great thing about the feeling of safety and trust is that it facilitates joint problem solving. If a staff member comes to your office and starts complaining, you can guide him or her by asking questions that might help him or her find the solution on his or her own. Genevieve, a nurse manager in an Alzheimer's unit, said that one staff member, Alvin, was in her office complaining about a lack of supplies. She said, "I just listened at first. I let him go on for what seemed like 10 minutes. He was complaining about the lack of supplies, how long they took to be delivered, and how long the problem had existed. I knew we were having problems, but didn't understand the depth of the issue."

Genevieve went on to say, "After Alvin calmed down, I complimented him on his commitment to the patients. I knew he would not be this upset if he did not care. I then asked him, 'If you could wave a magic wand, what would you want the solution to the supply problem to be?'" Alvin discussed improving the supply process, and some of his ideas made a lot of sense. Genevieve set up an appointment with the distribution department and invited Alvin to participate. His passion and great ideas were heard, his sense of trust with Genevieve increased, and some of the ideas were adopted (which led to better patient care). And it all started with an open door.

Closing the Open Door

The idea of an open door policy is metaphorical—meaning that you are open to talk with staff when they need you. However, sometimes the actual door needs to be closed. When a staff member is venting or sharing confidential information, it's perfectly fine to get up and close the door. Even someone who wants to share a good laugh can be disruptive to others depending on how close your office it to direct patient care areas. Be mindful that you can always invite staff in, and then close the door.

An open door invites staff in and provides the opportunity for them to engage with you in a nonthreatening environment. Some managers worry that staff will interrupt them at all hours if they have an open door policy, but most managers find that over time the need for the open-door diminishes because problems are addressed and staff do not feel the need to vent quite so much. Open your door and invite employees in—on their terms—and see what you learn. What a great way to create and build relationships.

Spending Time with Staff

The following comments are from nurses who were asked on a survey, "What should your nurse manager start doing?"

- "Come work with me once in a while."
- "Know what I do so you can help me better."
- "Understand what it is I am talking about when we talk about issues."

Several nurses shared their frustration about a lack of nurse manager face time in the work area. For example, "Start being more willing to help out when we are having a really busy day on the floor—even just with little things. If she (the manager) hears an IV pump beeping, she'll look for a nurse to turn it off. If the phone's ringing, she'll find someone to answer it. Pitching in to help out so our day is a little easier would make a huge difference!"

Like it or not, perception is reality when it comes to this touchy issue of spending time in your department. Scrubs or a suit? Will you be tracking down meds and answering phones or spending time in meetings and your office? The best answer is probably "All of the above!"

So what's a busy nurse manager to do? More and more managers are responsible for the financial side of their department (including monthly reconciliation, budgeting, meetings with finance, and so on). At the same time, you need to participate in organization-wide committees and attend leadership meetings. This is where the old adage about the quality—not the quantity—of your time comes into play. Effective nurse managers consistently spend time in their departments on all shifts, but not necessarily for long periods. There is no magic amount of time that good managers spend—you'll know it when you reach it.

I am not suggesting that you have to put on a uniform and take a patient load—although some managers do report working on a per-diem basis to keep their clinical skills up-to-date. That's for you to decide based on your personal goals, commitment to clinical practice, support from nursing leadership, and so forth. You do need to stay up-to-date on the challenges your staff face. If you are not familiar with the latest medication, procedural, or surgical issues your staff are dealing with, you will quickly lose your credibility, and the relationships will suffer.

Walk a Mile in My Shoes

On my national survey, when asked, "What else does the surveyor need to know?" one nurse shared, "I know it's not always possible, but I really wish our manager would, even for just a couple of hours, work on the floor to really understand what it's like. She seems out of touch with the stress and time constraints of the floor nurses, [and this] creates a distance between herself and her staff. We never feel like she understands what we're going through." Remember those famous words: walk a mile in my shoes, because that is what your staff members want you to do.

Hotko (2004), writing on behalf of the Studer Group, describes a process they have dubbed "Rounding for Outcomes," which complements our discussion of spending time with staff. Rounding for outcomes is the consistent practice of asking specific questions of key stakeholders—leaders, employees, physicians, and patients—to obtain actionable information.

The focus of questioning during rounding is to

- Build relationships.
- Harvest "wins" to learn what is going well, what is working, and who has been helpful.
- Identify process improvement areas.
- Repair and monitor systems to ensure chronic issues have been resolved.
- Ensure that key behavior standards in the organization are hardwired (or being consistently executed) to reward those who are following the standards and coach those who are not. To learn more, refer to *How to Increase Employee Retention and Drive Higher Patient Satisfaction*, by Barbara Hotko, R.N., M.P.A., Studer Group Coach (www.studergroup.com).

This idea of rounding for nurse managers certainly isn't new. In focus groups I conducted, managers shared that rounding is commonly used to address the desired outcomes of the department and to create a positive connection with their direct reports

---

Questions to Ask

Not sure what to say when you are rounding? Here's a partial listing of some questions to ask from the Studer Group:

- How is your family? Did your daughter graduate last week?
- Are there any physicians I need to recognize today?
- What systems can be working better?
- Do you have the tools and equipment to do your job? How long did it take you to find an IV pump today?

www.StuderGroup.com

When asked about how they juggle spending time in their departments, several nurse managers shared that they schedule these times in their calendars as appointments. If you wait until after you've scheduled everything else, and hope to find time to connect with staff, you will never find time. Start with your standing meetings, and then pencil in time for rounding. If geography cooperates, make a point of walking through your department on your way back from meetings so that you get a quick look at how things are going.

Peters and Waterman, in their 1982 business classic *In Search of Excellence*, dubbed this practice MBWA (Management By Wandering Around). Although written almost three decades ago, the practice is alive and well with managers who embrace the Partnership Protocol. When nurses are asked, "What should your nurse manager continue to do?" responses include the following:

- Be present on the unit and answer pages when she isn't.
- Work together side by side with us.
- Care for the nurses and patients.

As we all know, little things add up to big things, and as Woody Allen once said, "Eighty percent of success is just showing up." An inspiring nurse manager shows up in her department every day.

Be There or Be Square

I mentioned earlier that some nurse managers fall into the trap of thinking "no news is good news," and that not being around conveys a message that everything is fine. One nurse clearly counters this idea and speaks for her colleagues when she says, "I enjoy that she [the nurse manager] walks through the unit everyday, always finding something that needs attention in order to improve our workplace environment. Whether it's calling environmental services and making sure things are cleaned or personally refilling our Purell dispensers." Employees notice whether you are there.

The employees might not thank you, and they may not even act like they appreciate you being there, but most agree that face time on the unit shows support. And everyone is looking for a little more support at work.

Encouraging Autonomy

In addition to wanting you to be around to provide support, feedback, and guidance, your staff wants autonomy. For our purposes, autonomy is providing people with the freedom to be active participants in their work. We all want independence and the freedom to make decisions about our schedule, work responsibilities, and relationships with co-workers. This is why shared governance is so popular in health care. When we have the ability to contribute to actions as well as outcomes, we are much more likely to buy into the overall process.

The opposite of autonomy is micromanaging. A micromanager is acutely particular about *how* things are done, as opposed to a manager who focuses on outcomes. Think about the expression "She can't see the forest for the trees." Sometimes well-meaning managers—especially newer managers—feel like they should get involved in every decision that is made. These folks lose sight of the big picture and focus too much on minutiae. This leads to frustration and resentment because experienced staff members feel that their skills are unrecognized or undervalued.

I am not suggesting that you go to the other extreme and adopt a noninterventional, laissez-faire attitude. I'm saying you should aim for someplace in-between. Nurses also complain when they feel their managers are not getting involved enough—especially when dealing with holding staff accountable for agreed upon behaviors. When asked, "What do you wish your nurse manager would stop doing?" one of the most common responses is "micromanaging," and second is "ignoring the disruptive behavior of staff members who refuse to do what is outlined in their job descriptions." Increased employee autonomy often leads to increased engagement across the department.

Keeping a Professional Distance

One of the hardest transitions is when you are promoted to a management position in the area where you were a staff nurse. I have heard story after story about "walking the tightrope" between being a friend and a supervisor. Let's get that one clear right now: The tough-love answer is that the folks who report to you are not your friends. Friends act as confidants, problem solvers, sounding boards, and truth tellers. Managers act as business coaches, mentors, and catalysts for achieving business results. See how the lists differ. In focus groups, experienced nurse managers often talk about being friendly versus being friends. They stress the importance of boundaries when forging relationships.

The Misfits

Tara, a nurse manager who was promoted almost a year ago, shared a story that illustrated the point of friendly versus friends. Tara had worked in the ICU for more than 8 years when she was promoted to nurse manager. She was thrilled. Her peers supported her promotion. She realized early on that it was going to be tough to maintain her friendships with staff members in her new role. She worked hard to create professional boundaries so that she could effectively lead without being influenced by these friendships.

The telling moment came when she was invited to one of the staff member's weddings. She arrived at the reception and looked for her table number. She realized that she had been placed with "the misfits" (those folks who weren't at a table reserved for any particular family or friends group). She smiled, sat down, and realized that she had indeed achieved a new milestone. As bittersweet as the table placement was, she felt good about her role as the manager.

Believe it or not, your direct reports understand that you have new responsibilities and that you cannot, for instance, share private details about other employees. Just imagine how you would feel if your boss talked about your peers to you. Wouldn't you assume he or she was saying things about you to them, as well? That puts everyone in an uncomfortable position.

We all create boundaries with co-workers through the conversations we have (and do not have). If employees who were your good buddies start to talk about other staff members, excuse yourself and get back to work. For the few closest co-workers, you might want to address the issue head on in one-on-one meetings. You might start the conversation with something like, "Denise, I want to talk about our friendship and how you see it playing out now that I'm your manager. What thoughts do you have?" Then you can work it out so that to the best of your ability, you both are as comfortable as possible with the boundaries you create and put in place.

When it comes to holding staff accountable for expected behaviors, the manager/employee boundary becomes very important. A nurse manager, Marsha, shared a conversation with me she had with a former co-worker soon after she was promoted. The employee was showing up late for work. Marsha sat down to meet with the tardy employee and said, "I like you and I like working with you. You know that you need to be at work every day on time. If you don't come to work on time, I'll have to let you go, and you know I don't want to do that. Please get here on time from now on." The employee smiled and said she was sorry and showed up on time after the conversation.

Forming new relationships with nurse manager peers is a great way to gain support and role model healthy work relationships. Find the other managers who share your vision and values and work together to positively influence the organization.

Summary

Nurses, like other professionals, want to have a positive relationship with their manager. You can create and build upon this desire by

- Maintaining an open-door policy.
- Spending time with staff.
- Respecting autonomy.
- Keeping a professional distance.

None of these practices requires complex skills. Instead, they each require planning, commitment, and consistency. Start small and you will see incremental improvements in each area day by day. Over time, you'll find that you have employees who are true partners and who are more engaged and inspired.

CHAPTER 11
Support Team Members

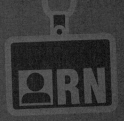

PARTNERSHIP PROTOCOL™

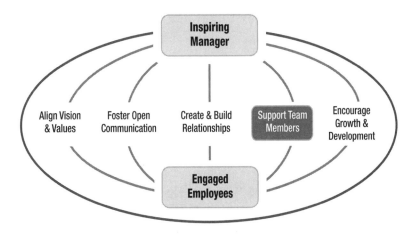

Most people agree that health care is a tough profession. The stress of experiencing life and death decision making on a regular basis takes its toll. Additionally, the pace of change is accelerating with updates to laws and regulations, technology advances, and pharmacology findings, to name but a few. No person can handle this alone; hence, the strong need for support among nurses and their co-workers.

You are probably not surprised to learn that 91% of the 196 nurses who responded to a national nursing survey rated "Building a strong team of co-workers" the number one action taken by managers that increases commitment, performance, and/or work effort of employees. Of nurse managers, 93.6% said the same thing. The top three responses regarding actions taken by nurse managers relate to team support. Everyone agrees that having a strong team is a key to success. The idea of working as a team is a foundational element of the Partnership Protocol.

In this chapter, I focus on what nurse managers must do to create and support strong teams:

- Understand the characteristics of effective teams.
- Create an atmosphere of trust with your staff.
- Offer fair and flexible scheduling.
- Ensure that the department's staffing is adequate.
- Provide satisfactory resources to meet departmental needs.

These categories bubbled up in the surveys and focus groups as well as in my experience working in health care. Before delving into the details, let's look at characteristics of effective teams.

Understanding the Characteristics of Effective Teams

The tendency of most busy managers is to focus on plans, actions, and outcomes. Unfortunately, with this focus, you can miss the underlying ideas that staff members have about teams in general and their team specifically. Plug into your team, and you'll learn volumes about their wants and needs for support. By "plug into," I mean bring up the idea of teamwork in discussions—both in one-on-one conversations and staff meetings—so that you better understand the beliefs and mindsets of your staff members. Ask questions about the team and listen as folks respond so that you understand the nuances of the team and its members.

In his best-selling book *The Five Dysfunctions of a Team*, Lencioni (2002) shares five key characteristics of dysfunctional teams. I have transferred the ideas from dysfunctional to functional for our use here. The traits of effective teams include the following:

- Trust
- Comfort with conflict
- Commitment
- Accountability
- Results focus

If you are especially interested in building your team, Lencioni's book is an easy read and full of great information. For now, my focus starts with a series of questions to ask to see how your team fares on the elements of supporting one another. Then you can determine the needed focus from there. I recommend that you ask these questions of yourself first and then in one-on-one meetings, small team meetings, and staff meetings. You also want to look at employee satisfaction data, patient satisfaction data, and quality indicators for further clues about your team's effectiveness.

Here are the questions:

- How do we build trust as a team on a daily basis? What trust issues does our team routinely deal with? How can I as a manager help to build trust?
- What kinds of conflicts arise in our department? What percentage of disagreements is taken underground and either ignored or talked about behind the staff member's back? What beliefs about conflict exist in staff members' minds?
- How do you and the staff demonstrate commitment to the team? Is commitment consistent or wavering? If wavering, what variables need to be addressed?
- Whose job is staff accountability? What tools do employees need in order to be better at holding each other accountable? How can you role model accountability more effectively?
- What results do you focus on? How are you incorporating a strategic connection in your messages about change? Do staff members recognize each other for a job well done? If not, why?

Once you've spent time delving into the answers to these questions, you will know which areas need work and which areas are going well. You may find that there is general consensus about the team, or you may find that opinions differ. Either way, the key action for you at this point is to focus on the team and its subtleties so that you can help them work more effectively together.

Time-Saver Tools
Team Survey

Using the questions listed, I've created a short survey you can give to staff members to get their anonymous feedback about team effectiveness (or lack thereof).

www.HiringFiringInspiring.com

The tricky part of teamwork on many nursing units is that the team changes with every shift. As a whole, you may find that the team meets the criteria discussed earlier, but one bad apple on a shift can throw off the whole team. Discussing these outliers is part of your job as a manager so that team members know their role in handling tough team situations. This is a process that takes time. Employees typically need to trust you before bonding occurs.

Creating an Atmosphere of Trust with Your Staff

To build a strong team, trust is vital, and it's an area completely within your control. Of 195 nurses who responded to a recent survey I conducted, 84.6% ranked "Creating an environment of trust within our unit/department" as strongly influencing their commitment, performance, and work effort. This was the third-highest ranking response. Wagner and Muller (2009) support this data in *Gallup Management Journal*. They wrote, "Trust is the linchpin of a partnership. With trust, both people can concentrate on their separate responsibilities, confident the other person will come through." Don't you agree that at the end of the day, we all want to be confident that the person who manages us will "come through?"

Fairness and Consistency

The number two influencer of commitment, performance, and work effort in the nursing survey mentioned previously was "Treating employees fairly and consistently" (87.6%). For some reason, maybe dating back to our younger days of sibling rivalry and playground scuffles, employees seem to worry and become irritated if they think that other staff members are being treated differently from them. Additionally, staff members seem to think that managers are not working as hard as nurses are. In another article, Wagner and Muller (2009) share, "When Gallup asked people whether they and their manager share the workload fairly between them, the answers tilted dramatically toward the negative end of the scale. Nearly one-third strongly disagreed. Only 16% strongly agreed." We're not here to figure out the psychology of this phenomenon, we just want to make sure that it doesn't cause added stress in your department.

Perceptions Count

To avoid the perception of unfairness, be transparent in your dealings with staff. However, I'm not suggesting that you make conversations with staff members public; confidentiality is a key to building trust. I am suggesting that you are fair in staffing and scheduling (especially with time off), fair in the way you communicate, fair in asking for input, fair in your support of staff, and so forth. One nurse in the survey articulated, "I wish my nurse manager would start listening and getting feedback from all staff … not just the whiny ones who e-mail her with tattling!"

Repeatedly in the survey, nurses complained about nurse managers who play favorites. Throughout the comments, favoritism is mentioned in a number of ways, including the following:

- Employees receiving special privileges.
- Communicating information to select people.
- Defending staff members who don't do their jobs.
- Saying yes to physicians without thinking about consequences to staff.

- Not holding everyone to the same standard.
- Speaking negatively about staff members to other staff members.

I think we all agree that these management behaviors are unproductive and uninspiring. Unfortunately, in the pressure of day-to-day management, it can be easy to fall into these traps (less-than-optimal management behaviors) if you are not paying attention. Perception plays a major role in a lot of these comments, so ask for feedback on your blind spots so that you aren't accused of playing favorites.

Fairness and Equity

One nurse in the survey said, "A good manager shows fairness and equity with all staff. Nurses respond in a positive manner when their manager will stand up for them and show general concern and support for their professional and personal growth and well-being. This isn't the way most business managers operate, but health care workers are another breed and need this personal support due to the type of work we do every day, which can be quite taxing on our emotions." Make fairness and equity a priority and watch as you build trust and teamwork through your actions.

When you have an idea of your team's trust level and perceptions, you can focus on other areas of support, including scheduling and staffing and resource management. Scheduling is the process you use for assigning work shifts, staffing involves having the right people (and enough of them) at work during a given shift, and effective resource management includes providing staff members who are working with the tools they need to complete their tasks successfully.

Offering Fair and Flexible Scheduling

Effectively scheduling staff is like putting together a puzzle. Depending on the type of department you manage, the number of staff needed, and the variability of the shifts, your scheduling puzzle could range from the 25-piece starter to the complex 1000-piece meadow. Let's continue using the metaphor of the puzzle to illustrate an effective format for scheduling. The format includes the following:

- Looking at the big picture.
- Putting together the border.
- Filling in the easy, middle pieces.
- Placing the final, tougher-to-fit pieces.

Looking at the Big Picture

The first step in putting together a puzzle is to look at the big picture. It's a good idea to study the cover of the puzzle box so that you can see the nuances of the picture, colors, and such. Remember that scheduling should align with the vision and values of your organization so that you and the staff can deliver on your desired internal brand. In the case of scheduling a nursing unit, the puzzle is usually a montage, with at least three pictures to consider. Picture one is the administrative area—including budget and finance considerations. Picture two is nursing practice—including safety, quality of care, laws, and regulations. Picture three is the staff and their desire for flexibility. Although it's challenging, as a nurse manager your job when creating the schedule is to balance all three parts of the big picture. The next three areas help with balancing the parts.

Putting Together the Border

When you put together a puzzle, you start with the border. That's the easy part. The pieces have a flat edge, so you can easily identify them. The same holds true for creating a schedule. Start with a framework. You know from past experience what coverage is needed in your department. Maybe in your area the framework includes 12-hour shifts with a few other shifts thrown into the mix. Or, perhaps you are in an outpatient area that has businesslike hours with one late night. These both are examples of frameworks.

The border is the predictable piece of the schedule. Look at trends to see what has worked in the past. During flu season, your scheduling needs might increase. During holidays, the pace might slow down depending on your clinical area. Get the picture? The framework for your scheduling acts as the border on your puzzle.

Caller ID: Friend or Foe?

A nurse manager shared this success story with me. [I work on] "really understanding my staff's scheduling needs/wants and trying to make it fit into the nursing unit's needs. The very visible efforts encouraged everyone to learn each others needs/wants and really made for team accountability in scheduling. Everyone worked together to create that ideal schedule, and in three years, I [the nursing manager] came in to cover staffing only once. The staff started answering their phones when they saw us calling and would usually come in if needed, instead of screening their calls and ignoring the potential needs of the unit."

An important piece of the framework is the process you use for creating the schedule. Self-scheduling is a popular option for creating the framework. Under a self-scheduling system, when staff see what the scheduling needs are for the unit and have an opportunity to fill in their desired times to work, they understand the big picture and feel more empowered to adequately staff the unit.

On the nursing staff survey, I asked, "What should your nurse manager continue to do?" Responses related to scheduling include the following:

- Establish creative, flexible scheduling.
- Accommodate schedules and provide for time off when requested.

- Allow self-scheduling (mentioned numerous times).
- Be open with schedules.
- Allow me to have a flexible work schedule.

The bottom line is that staff members appreciate flexible scheduling because they all have lives outside of work.

Filling In the Easy, Middle Pieces

The full-time staff that you assign to work a certain schedule represent the easy, middle pieces of the puzzle. Because of an aging nursing workforce, flexible scheduling is important. One nursing supervisor I interviewed said, "I just can't work 12-hour shifts anymore … it's too much." The baby boomers want fewer 12-hour shifts, but younger generations often appreciate being able to work three 12-hour shifts to have time for other interests the rest of the week. Listen to what staff has to say and try to be as flexible as possible.

Scheduling the Generations

I'm sure you've discovered that having folks from several generations in the workplace can be challenging. They all want to have input when it comes to creating the schedule. If you are feeling the pull of Gen Y versus Gen X versus Baby Boomers, hold meetings with your staff members to brainstorm creative scheduling ideas.

Use the traffic light format again and ask these questions to get a conversation going:

1. What should we stop doing related to scheduling?
2. What should we continue doing?
3. What should we start doing?

Ask for a few volunteers (optimally, from diverse generations) to form a committee to provide follow up for all the ideas presented, and then follow through on the recommendations.

You count on your "middle pieces"—those employees who consistently come to work and do a great job. Don't ignore their requests. You want to support them with their scheduling concerns. One respondent to my survey said, "Be more flexible with our schedules. We are required to pick vacation time in January. Obtaining a day not submitted at that time is usually denied." This rigidity is very disengaging. On the opposite side of the spectrum, another nurse wrote, "My manager realizes that our home lives impact our work performance, and she attempts to give us our schedule requests if possible." She wants the manager to continue this behavior. If you want your regular staff to continue to fill in the scheduling puzzle, flexibility is key.

Placing the Final, Tougher-to-Fit Pieces

Have you done one of those puzzles with a background that is all one color? These pieces are particularly tough to fill in because no distinct elements offer guidance for the placement. This same phenomenon holds true when trying to fill in the gaps in your schedule. Using per diem and agency staff is expensive. Most mangers I speak with have shrinking budgets, so a heavy use of outside staff negatively affects the unit financially. Overtime is another budget drain, so consistent scheduling is important on all fronts.

Based on feedback I received, the best solution to this problem is having a group of engaged, invested employees who feel responsible for making sure the schedule is realistic and works well over time.

Employees Appreciate Flexibility

Connie, RN, DON, shared this great suggestion in one of my surveys: "I practice very flexible scheduling. I tell my staff regularly that I recognize that they have commitments at home, and if they tell me ahead of time, I will do everything to grant their requests. I don't use agency staff, and therefore count heavily on the staff coming to work as scheduled. The staff really appreciated this effort to honor their requests, even on short notice, and have rallied by working for each other and often they have covered themselves. They also do not work 'short.' We do everything, including RNs, LPNs, DONs, working when we have a spot we cannot cover. This does a lot for retention of staff and resident and family satisfaction. I also follow the attendance policy of our facility and will terminate a staff member for poor attendance. This also works for retention and staff morale, as I don't have a lot of call-offs and everyone is treated fairly."

People like control. Most people find controlling their work schedule helps them to enjoy work more because they have fewer conflicts with events outside of work. When employees can balance personal commitments with work scheduling, stress decreases and performance improves. Master the art of solving the schedule puzzle and you will see positive results.

Ensuring That the Department's Staffing Is Adequate

I'm sure this won't come as a surprise to you: When asked what keeps them up at night, nearly three-quarters of the 44 survey responses that nurse managers provided included *staffing*. As I mentioned earlier, for our purposes here, staffing involves having the right people (and enough of them) at work during a given shift. Health care staffing is a contentious issue based on patient acuity, budgets, and safety concerns. According to M. W. Stanton (2004) in the *Agency for Healthcare Research and Quality,* "Hospitals with low nurse staffing levels tend to have higher rates of poor patient outcomes, such as pneumonia, shock, cardiac arrest, and urinary tract infections. Complementing those studies is a number of other studies addressing the growing nurse workload and rising rates of burnout and job dissatisfaction."

Getting the right employees in the right spot doing the right job is a balancing act based on your census and patient acuity, the diversity of skill sets and experience, and your financial budget. My focus here when it comes to staffing is on what is directly within your control.

An element of staffing within your control is the competency level of the staff. If the nurses and ancillary staff are not properly trained and competency tested, the issue becomes quality—as well as quantity. One nurse manager I spoke with brought up the issue of poorly trained and underutilized patient care techs. She said that the nurses were afraid to delegate to the techs because of their attitudes and lack of skill. The manager jumped in to address the problem by focusing on quality and quantity, and the staffing issues decreased.

Look at Quality *and* Quantity

If you feel like some employees in your department are not working up to their potential, it is time to jump in. Additionally, support those staff members who are performing to standards. Nurses report frustration when others aren't doing their jobs and the nurse manager doesn't step in to solve the problem. Try these steps to get started:

1. Contact the clinical education department (or advanced practice nurse who supports your department) and ask for help with competency validation.

2. Review the job descriptions of all staff members—are they up-to-date and realistic? If not, ask for help from star performers and HR to update the job descriptions.

3. Create a plan for competency validation using staff members and education staff (either on the job or in lab simulations).

4. Communicate the plan.

5. Implement the competency testing.

6. Offer training for staff members who do not meet expectations. Offer your nursing staff training on delegating properly. (Go to your state board of nursing website for current information about effective delegation.)

7. Hold staff accountable for completing all aspects of their job.

When all is said and done, having all staff members performing the desired skills is like adding people to the mix without adding to the cost.

Talking about staffing issues with your high performers will give you insight into their concerns and suggestions. Because the foundation of being an inspiring manager is partnership, sharing the problem solving with others will broaden your possibilities. Staff members often have a different perspective from you as a manager; hearing that perspective can be very helpful. Challenges that you don't know about can be uncovered via open dialogue about staffing. If asked, staff members often have creative solutions for staffing problems. Another idea is to work collaboratively with other nurse managers to learn best practices for filling staffing gaps. In the case of problem solving about staffing, the old saying two heads are better than one definitely rings true.

Providing Satisfactory Resources to Meet Departmental Needs

In addition to people, every nursing department depends on a vast array of resources to keep it running. From the physical plant (floors, air conditioning, heat, and so on), equipment, and supplies for education and training, your job is to support staff, remove roadblocks, and pave the way for excellent care delivery.

To provide this type of support, you need to be in the department on a regular basis. When you are in the department, be sure to focus on these needs. If you do so, the staff will see that you care about their ability to get the job done.

To help alleviate and solve resource problems, you'll want to form relationships with staff from other departments who are able to assist you. As clinicians, nurse managers often think about clinical areas (for example, radiology, pharmacy, or the lab). However, do not forget nonclinical areas, such as distribution and information technology. To form relationships with these managers, set up a meet and greet with your peer from the other department when there are no identified problems. Make a list of the departments you support and those that support you. And remember folks in human resources and nursing education; they are resource partners, too. Work through your list, meeting and greeting and establishing relationships that you can nurture and call on later when necessary.

After all, cultivating relationships with those in the departments you work with frequently will make life much easier when something goes wrong.

What Do I Say?

When you meet with your peers from the various departments that support your area, try these conversation starters and listen carefully to the responses. Feel free to take notes so that you don't forget, and dig deeper, as appropriate.

- What do you do in your department?
- How did you end up working in this area?
- What suggestions do you have for our two areas working together more effectively?
- How should I handle a problem if one arises?
- Is there anything else I need to know or something that you need from me?

Time-Saver Tools
Meet & Greet Cheat Sheet

Print out this cheat sheet and take it when you meet with your peers from other departments. Just think how organized you'll feel (and look).

www.HiringFiringInspiring.com

When it comes to resources, supporting the team means being a liaison and advocate for the employees to other departments. When you provide the staff with the tools they need to do their job, they are able to get their job done more easily and they feel less stressed and more productive.

Supply and Demand

Remember the story of Alvin and Genevieve from Chapter 10, "Create and Build Relationships?" Alvin, a GNA, frustrated because of a lack of supplies in his work area, was complaining to his manager, Genevieve, about the challenges and the resulting poor patient care. Genevieve listened to Alvin's venting and worked on solving the problem. She stepped up to the plate in a support role and set up a meeting with the distribution department to iron out the difficulties. Alvin was happy, his co-workers appreciated the efforts, and best of all, the patients benefited from the right supplies being available for their care. Genevieve could have passed along the responsibility to Alvin, but instead she showed support for the team as she intervened and ultimately worked with everyone to solve the problem.

Summary

According to nearly 200 nurses who responded to a national survey, building a strong team of co-workers is the most influential action you can take to increase staff commitment, performance, and work effort. When commitment, performance, and work effort increase, the patient reaps the rewards. When patients are satisfied, the organization does well. To build a strong health care team, management must

- Understand characteristics of effective teams.
- Create an atmosphere of trust.
- Offer fair and flexible scheduling.
- Ensure that the department's staffing is adequate.
- Provide satisfactory resources for meeting departmental needs.

Supporting team members creates a strong team, a strong department, and ultimately, a strong organization. The stronger your team is, the more effective you are as a leader. Go, Team!

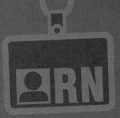

CHAPTER 12
Encourage Growth and Development

PARTNERSHIP PROTOCOL™

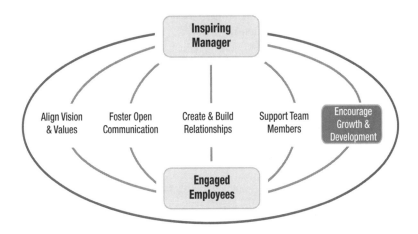

A key element of the Partnership Protocol for inspiring staff is employee growth and development. As a nurse manger, you have many opportunities to influence this area. From providing on-the-job training to inviting staff to attend national conferences, you are sending important messages about professional development. The first hurdle is providing employees with the chance to use their talents. After that, you are charged with offering ongoing opportunities for formal and informal growth and development.

According to the Blessing White *2008 Employee Engagement Report*, "More than half (53%) of employees want to use their unique capabilities to [do what they do best] each day or move their career and growth forward [career development opportunities and training]." The opposite—feeling stagnant in your job—is very disengaging. When employees feel bored or uninspired, they often cost the organization untold dollars in lost productivity, mistakes, and patient dissatisfaction. You can increase staff engagement and the partnership mindset in your department by exploring personal or professional growth opportunities with them.

I had the pleasure of working in a hospital education department for almost seven years. During that time, I was happy to confirm that most people enjoy expanding their knowledge, skills, and abilities at work if it's done at a manageable pace. This made my education job extremely rewarding. I found that patient care staff learn and grow though many avenues, including the following:

- The work itself
- On-the-job training
- In-house training
- Conferences
- Higher education
- Certification and virtual training

As a manager, you have the opportunity (and responsibility) to provide a variety of opportunities for growth and development. My focus here is on nursing; however, you can apply these same concepts to all staff members in your department.

Play to Their Strengths

When I worked in staff development for a community teaching hospital, my manager, Liz, was good at providing me with opportunities to do what I do best. When I got bored with the routine part of my job, she asked me what my other interests were. I shared that I would like to be involved in more hospital-wide projects so that I could have more of an impact and get to know more people throughout the organization. When a Missing Wheelchair Quality Improvement team needed input from the education department, Liz invited me to be a part of the team. I'm sure she was secretly happy because it was one less meeting for her to attend. I loved learning about the quality improvement process and meeting others. We both benefited because she focused on my growth and development.

The Work Itself

What makes work meaningful? Fortunately, the answer differs for each of us. If it were the same for everyone, then we would all want to do the same job and it would be tough to get the work of health care done. Sometimes managers get so busy that they forget about connecting work and meaning, or purpose. In my book *SHIFT to Professional Paradise*, I share tools and tips for becoming the Chief Paradise Officer (CPO) of your job. A CPO is satisfied, energized, and productive. Utilizing your strengths is a precursor to being the CPO of your job. Growth and development is one avenue to get there.

As health care workers, we often assume that people choose their jobs because of the meaning they find in the tasks they engage in, but this assumption isn't always true. Over time, meaning gets lost in the everyday challenges of work, and people forget the pull they felt when they first started their careers. For health care employees, the work itself can be intense and cause burnout over time. As a manager, you are in a great position to help employees reconnect with their passion at work.

Recognizing and Engaging Staff Strengths

Buckingham and Clifton, in their best-selling book *Now, Discover Your Strengths* (2001), write extensively about the value of strengths-based work. Through their work with the Gallup Organization, they found that when employees are using their key strengths, they produce better outcomes. As a manager, do you know the strengths of your staff? And are you providing work opportunities to capitalize on these strengths? If not, you may be missing out on opportunities for growth and development.

Employees who are finding meaning and are engaged at work have a *positive* attitude, an *intense* connection, and *exert* extra effort. I call this their PIE. Here's an exercise to help employees find their PIE in the Sky™. I call this exercise finding your PIE in the Sky because you are asking staff members to assign percentages that reflect an "if they could have it any way" mindset. This works well at a staff meeting or in one-on-one discussions.

1. Share an illustration of something that motivates you (for example, making a positive connection with others), and then ask employees to write down 3 or 4 things that motivate them at work. What do they do at work that puts a skip in their step? Common responses include making a difference, problem solving, teamwork, learning new things, and helping others.

2. Ask the employees to assign percentages to each motivator from the list to create a total of 100%. The percentage is based on what part of the day they would like to spend doing this responsibility (in a perfect world).

3. Ask employees to draw a large circle on a piece of paper and make a PIE chart with the percentages (see Figure 12.1).

4. Ask employees to discuss their largest piece of the PIE and why it is important to them. Invite people to share their response publicly so that everyone knows about each other's motivators.

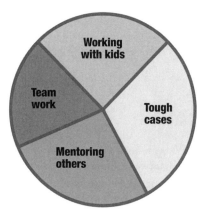

Figure 12.1

When you know the biggest segments of the PIE, you can

- Make assignments based on them.
- Invite the person to participate in educational sessions or meetings as they relate to the areas of interest.
- Include a plan for expanding knowledge, skills, and abilities in these areas in performance appraisal meetings.

Jody's PIE in the Sky

Jody, a nurse working in the ED, shared her PIE in the Sky with her manager, Stacey. The conversation was illuminating for both of them. Based on her responses, Stacey talked with Jody about precepting new nurses in the pediatric ED. She also worked to include Jody in tough cases when it made sense. Because Stacey knows the big pieces of Jody's PIE, she can connect her with what matters most to her and, therefore, provide a more engaging work environment. Jody has a renewed sense of what she enjoys about her work, and this is contagious to co-workers and patients. Stacey and Jody could sit back and enjoy that slice of PIE in the Sky.

An interesting part about inviting staff to share their PIE in the Sky with each other is that team members can invite folks to work with them on projects that meet the criteria. This provides a "win-win" for everyone.

On-the-Job Training

Employees are always learning from their co-workers. Sometimes the learning is positive and other times not so positive. This is called social learning theory. According to Raymond A. Noe (2005), in his book *Employee Training and Development*, "Social learning theory emphasizes that people learn by observing other persons whom they believe are credible and knowledgeable." Staff members typically figure out who they think are "credible and knowledgeable," and then they model their behaviors. This points to the need for a strong team of credible and knowledgeable staff members because people are learning from each other all the time.

The Real World

In my days of presenting new employee orientation at a large community teaching hospital, I regularly shared information about how important patient satisfaction was to the institution. Through interactive exercises, the staff learned the techniques for creating great first impressions and handling difficult customers.

I was disappointed to overhear an experienced nurse in one department tell a new hire, "That's all well and good, but here in the real world, we don't worry about all that. We do the best we can, and if the patient is satisfied, that's a bonus."

As a manager, always remember that saying it doesn't make it so. Employees need to see others demonstrating the desired behaviors and ultimately experiencing the positive consequences; learning on the job is a key component of this. Therefore, your job of holding staff accountable becomes more important than ever.

As a manager, you are in a great position to encourage productive social learning. Asking experienced staff to mentor less-experienced staff shows the veterans that you are confident in their knowledge, skills, and abilities. Because budgets do not always include enough money for external growth and development opportunities, peer mentoring is a great way to accomplish two goals: Staff members learn new skills from other team members, and the team members doing the teaching feel good about their contribution.

In-House Training

Depending on where you work, employees may have access to in-house training programs offered by the staff-development department. In a focus group with nurses, one nurse complained about mandatory training. She said, "My manager makes too many things mandatory." When I asked her more about this, she shared that she wasn't interested in all the mandatory training (like compliance or safety training) and that she wanted to attend more clinical training. As a manager, you are charged with creating compelling reasons for staff to attend (and participate in) all training. Work with the education department to help you with marketing the message about the programs to improve participation.

On the other hand, you want to be an advocate for training opportunities for staff in areas that they identify as important. Is there a new procedure, medication, or piece of technology that the staff wants to learn more about? Having a strong relationship with the advanced practice nurses and educators will help pave the way for more staff training. Sometimes all it takes is making the request.

If you work in a smaller facility that doesn't have an in-house education department, you'd be surprised how much free or low-cost information is available on the Internet. Go back to the PIE in the Sky exercise and see who has "mentoring or coaching others" or "learning new things" as one of their big pieces of the PIE.

Ask this person to lead a training program on a selected topic. Encourage him or her to use up-to-date resources (the local library, Internet, nursing associations, and so on) to create a short training program for the staff. You can provide guidance and review the materials to make sure he or she is on target.

On the day of the program, introduce your "guest speaker" and recognize his or her hard work of putting together the program. After the session, ask the staff for feedback and share it with the presenter so he or she knows what was learned and where he or she needs to improve. In this case, you are helping someone achieve their PIE in the Sky, and their co-workers are learning at the same time. That's called using your resources wisely.

I Can't Handle Another Job!

Feeling overwhelmed at the idea of creating in-services for staff? That's easy. Share the responsibility. You don't have to do this yourself. Try this at your next staff meeting. (All you need is a flipchart or board to write on.)

1. Explain that a new agenda item for staff meetings is going to be "Professional Growth and Development." Ask people to share topics they would like to learn more about and write the ideas on the flipchart.

2. Ask people to identify what associations they belong to or attend meetings for. Make a list on another piece of flipchart paper.

3. In groups of 2 or 3 people, ask the staff to brainstorm ideas for providing professional growth and development for staff on specific topics. (You can split up the topics to make this step easier.) These ideas can include internal and external resources.

4. Have each group report their ideas and record those on another piece of flipchart paper.

5. Prioritize the list and select the first topic. Ask for a few volunteers to be in charge of putting together the in-service.

Continue the process each month (or every other month) at staff meetings and watch the employees grow and develop.

Regardless of whether you have internal education resources, you have the responsibility to provide training for employees. Sometimes that just means being a conduit for the information. In a survey one nurse said, "My nurse manager should start informing staff of development/CEU (Continuing Education Unit) opportunities, realizing that this is an important aspect of nursing, not just staffing the area." Other times, providing training means finding your own internal resources for conducting the training. The good news is that resources abound in health care if you make a point to look for them.

Conferences

If you search the Internet for *nursing associations,* hundreds appear. One of the selling points of these organizations is their opportunity for continuing-education, through either conferences or the use of technology. You can select from broad groups like the American Nurses Association or specialist groups like the Society for Vascular Nursing. Visitors are usually welcome at their meetings, so membership is not generally necessary.

Pick a few associations that make sense for your staff and ask for volunteers to attend a few local meetings and report back on the value of attending. Because many states and nursing disciplines require continuing education credits so that the staff members stay current in their chosen field, the associations provide low-cost CEU sessions. Ideally, you will have budget dollars to use for sending staff members for training at conferences. If you do, make sure you spread the wealth and let a variety of employees attend. Having an application process can streamline your decision making about whom to send. Let employees ask to go, instead of you just picking who should attend. The application process may minimize feelings of favoritism that staff might have.

Conference Application

Creating an application for staff members to complete to attend a conference can feel like a lot of work. Here's one you can use:

1. Demographics: name, contact information.
2. What conference would you like to attend?
3. What are the costs associated with attending (include registration fees, travel, etc.)?
4. How many hours/days of work will be involved?
5. What are three key things you would like to learn at the conference?
6. How will you share this information with other staff members?
7. What else do I need to know about you attending this conference?

Just type up these questions and ask staff members to fill out the application. You can make the decision about who goes or create a Growth and Development Team that decides how to allocate budget dollars. Make sure you spend the money and document the benefits of conference attendance in case you need it for future budget discussions.

Many managers ask employees who attend a conference to review what they learned with others. This is good for the attendee (because it reinforces the key learning) as well as for those who do not attend. Ask the person to set up the in-service, publicize it, and present the new information. Ask someone to take minutes, or better yet, videotape the program so those who can't attend will eventually benefit as well.

Conferences provide a fabulous opportunity for growth and development through formal training sessions, but they are also great for informal networking. This networking is another important part of growth because it expands the person's view of the world and provides perspective that you just can't get working in your own facility. Some nurse managers worry that their staff members will find greener pastures if they are networking outside of the facility. If you are doing a great job, the opposite will be true. Your staff will see how great you are to work for and how well your organization supports them.

Higher Education

Some employees want to grow and develop through higher education. Many nurses would like the opportunity to get their bachelor of science in nursing (BSN), and ancillary staff might want to go to nursing school. Does your organization have tuition reimbursement? If so, invite someone from the human resources department to attend one of your staff meetings to talk about this important benefit. Encourage employees to pursue higher education and keep track of their progress through informal conversations.

How Was School Today?

When I was in graduate school working on my master's degree in human resource development, I worked in the staff development department at the hospital. I will always remember how supportive my manager (and her boss) where of my studies. Each of them showed interest in what I was learning and asked how I could better apply that learning on the job to benefit the institution and myself.

If you know that one of your employees is taking college classes, be sure to offer support and encouragement by checking in on his or her progress. Depending on the course of study at the time, he or she could present the latest information on a relevant topic to team members at an in-service (either virtually or in-person).

Because many higher education institutions are tailoring their programs to working adults, you'll want to offer as much flexibility in scheduling as you can so that staff members can meet their education requirements. Without playing favorites or breaking your own scheduling rules, work with the employee to provide a schedule that allows for classroom time and clinical rotations. This will pay off in the long run through retention. Most employees recognize and appreciate this flexibility, and it reinforces their decision to work for you at your organization long after the degree is completed.

Certification and Virtual Training

Getting certified is another method of growth and development for health care employees. Depending on the area in which you manage, there is most likely some type of national certification that staff can achieve. When you visit www.nursecredentialing. org, open the Certification tab to see the broad range of specialty areas. From cardiovascular to pediatric to psychiatric nursing, the requirements are listed, as are study guides for testing.

Finally, virtual training is the newest frontier for growth and development. Simply type *continuing education for nurses* into your Internet search engine and more than 2 million links appear. According to www.nursecredentialing.org, the American Nurses Credentialing Center (ANCC) "is the world's leading accreditor of continuing nursing education (CNE). Anytime you take a continuing education course in your nursing career, you should check that it is accredited by ANCC so that you can be certain it is a quality course that meets all required standards for your certification, licensing, and other purposes." The Honor Society of Nursing, Sigma Theta Tau International Website, at http://www.nursingsociety.org/ offers free continuing education opportunities. Just click on the Education link. At the Nurseceu.com Website, there are more than 40 different nursing specialties with clickable links to specific CEU workshops for minimal fees.

As you can see, there is no shortage of opportunities for staff members to keep their knowledge levels current. Showing your support for this learning lets staff members know that you value their growth and development.

Summary

Do your best to be an advocate for the staff (including all employees—not just nurses) so that they feel valued. When people learn and grow, they are more engaged, and this leads to improved patient outcomes. According to Stuart Crandell (2009) in *Talent Management* magazine, "Talented people often leave because they are in roles they do not find rewarding, when a fairly simple job redesign can make the roles more attractive."

Include employee growth and development in your plans for inspiring employees, and you'll see the quality of patient care get better, employee morale improve, and your important metrics increase. It is definitely worth your investment (both time and budgetary). Make sure you stay on track for growth and development yourself. Reading this book is a great start!

CHAPTER 13
Take Care of Yourself

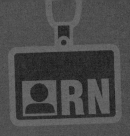

PARTNERSHIP PROTOCOL™

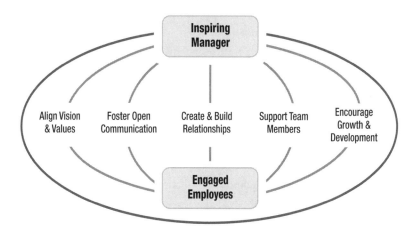

Congratulations! You've successfully navigated the five key elements of the Partnership Protocol:

- Align vision and values.
- Foster open communication.
- Create and build relationships.
- Support team members.
- Encourage growth and development.

You have learned about many tools and techniques for engaging staff members in your department. As an inspiring manager, your focus has been on others and your role in helping your team at work. Now the focus turns to you and your ability to take care of yourself.

Imagine that you are going on a well-deserved vacation. You have just boarded the plane for some tropical destination. As your airplane gets ready for take off, the flight attendants give instructions about what to do if a disaster strikes while you are on the plane. One of the most important announcements is to put on your own oxygen mask first, then help others put on theirs. The same premise holds true for nursing managers. You must inspire and take care of yourself before you can hope to inspire others. This isn't being selfish—it's a matter of survival. If you want to be inspired *and* inspiring, you must take care of yourself. Otherwise, just like the airplane, you will crash and burn.

In this chapter, I focus on the following five main areas of self-care:

- Maximizing your time at work.
- Remembering life outside of work.
- Engaging in professional development.
- Working with your boss.
- Finding a mentor.

Each of these areas provides an avenue of self-care that will help you to maintain your momentum (and sanity) as a manager. The job of a nurse manager is definitely not a sprint; it's a marathon (or even a triathlon) that requires preparation, endurance, and a mighty will to succeed.

Maximizing Your Time at Work

The way you choose to spend your time at work has a lot to do with taking care of yourself. I'm sure there are days when your schedule feels very reactive and somewhat out of control. This leads to increased stress, decreased energy, and less-than-stellar results. The best approach is to focus on what is within your control and manage the rest. Begin by meeting with your boss to talk specifically about your schedule and how you spend your time when you are at work.

To start this conversation with your boss, focus on the strategic business objectives you are working on. Ask your boss to confirm the top 3 or 4 priorities for your area. Now, look at how and where you spend your time. With your boss, answer the following questions:

- Do your actions line up with the priorities?
- What appointments or items on your to-do list could be rearranged or delegated to others?
- What items should be dropped altogether?
- What actions or appointments should be added?
- What are realistic expectations for responding to email and voicemail messages?
- What resources do you have available for delegating tasks?
- What else do you notice about how you spend your time?

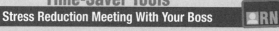

Time-Saver Tools
Stress Reduction Meeting With Your Boss

If you are feeling stressed at work, ask for help. Use this meeting template as a guide for talking with your boss..
www.HiringFiringInspiring.com

After you have a clearer picture of how you spend your time at work, you can brainstorm and problem-solve to reallocate your time if that's what's needed. Because you did this exercise with your manager, he or she better understands your typical days and can help you by running interference with others, supporting your decisions with staff, and so forth. For great ideas on how to be more productive at work, visit ProductiveDay.com and click the News and Resources link for helpful articles by productivity expert, Leslie Shreve.

Stop the Meeting Mania

One complaint I hear repeatedly from staff members and managers is the excessive number of meetings they must attend. Meetings often create a scheduling conflict with other important aspects of your day, including the following:

- Spending informal time in your department.
- Patient and staff rounding.
- Meeting with staff one-on-one.

When you review how you spend your time at work with your manager, discuss how meetings impact your day. And follow the suggestions in this sidebar to decrease time spent in meetings.

First, make a list of the following:

- Standing meetings you attend.
- Meetings that pop up at the last minute.
- Meetings you schedule.
- Organization-wide meetings.

For each meeting, ask yourself the following:

- What is the desired or real outcome of me attending this meeting?
- Do I really need to go to this meeting?
- Is there someone else who could go in my place?
- Who do I need to talk with about not going?

Another idea is to suggest 50-minute meetings throughout the organization, or at least in your department, so that you have time to check e-mail, visit the restroom, or stop by your unit between meetings. This way, you can catch your breath and focus on what is happening next.

Regardless of what you decide to do, spending time focusing on how you spend your time at work will create an increased sense of control, which is one step on the journey to taking care of yourself. The other benefits are that staff will see more of you, you'll have time to provide real-time compliments and coaching, and you will be an excellent role model for staff when they schedule their time in your department.

Remembering Life Outside of Work

I realize that this is a book about managing at work, but there comes a time when it's necessary to talk about your time outside of work because of its impact on your professional life. A term that is bandied about in stress management circles is *work/life balance*. Do you believe there is such a thing as work/life balance? The word "balance" conjures up a scale with two sides being equal. I think that for most people, our work life and our personal life rarely balance because we spend a vast majority of our waking hours working. Imbalance, in terms of literal hours spent on each activity, isn't really the issue for most people. Perhaps a more appropriate word to describe the goal here is "complementary," as in, your personal life complements your professional life and vice versa.

One of the best things about work is the meaning that we find in our professional responsibilities. For many people, work provides an identity, a sense of purpose, and a contribution, or making a difference. I know from my conversations with nurse managers that most feel the same way. Your work is a calling, not just a job, and as such provides many payoffs beyond a paycheck.

The problem is that many nurse managers feel called to their jobs to the point that they have a hard time pulling away; after all, the work is never done. They worry that something will fall through the cracks, so work stays on their minds more than it should. On a recent survey one nurse wisely commented, "I wish my nurse manager would stop spending all her waking hours at work or answering the phone after she leaves. Honestly, she is a 24/7 nurse, and that is way beyond the scope of healthy for us and especially her."

How does the conscientious nurse manager disengage? First, you need to train others to fill in for you when you are gone so that you can relax. The worst position to be in at work is to be indispensable. Your ego might like the idea of being needed all the time, but your body and soul crave some downtime and separation from the stressors of work.

The 3 Ds of Spare Time

Outside interests and hobbies that captivate you in your spare time help you handle stress at work. Are you laughing at the idea of "spare" time, thinking about the 24/7 nature of your work and all your other obligations? Read on for suggestions.

What do you like to do when you're not at work? Don't remember having spare time? Well, as you know from work, the squeaky wheel gets the grease. Make finding spare time to take care of yourself a "squeaky wheel" by asking for help from others at work and at home. Here are the 3 Ds:

- **Delegate:** Many nurses are poor at delegating (at home and at work). The idea of giving control to someone else makes us nervous. Let that notion go. Share the work—someone else will learn and grow if you let them (and yes, children are good at chores if you don't look too closely).

- **Daydream:** Soak in the tub, take a walk, or talk with a friend and daydream about what you would do with your free time if you had any. Visualize how you would spend the time. Use your senses, be specific, and picture yourself in the daydream.

- **Do it:** Leave work. Hand off your phone or beeper to someone else. Start knitting, salsa dancing, and watching your kids at sporting events or piano practice. Take the flying leap and leave work. Let someone else be in charge. Just do it!

You wouldn't expect your staff members to be at work all the time. Why do you expect it of yourself? Being a positive role model includes taking time away from work to relax and recharge. Remember, you need to be inspired before you can inspire others.

Engaging in Professional Development

In Chapter 12, "Encourage Growth and Development," I discussed the need to provide growth and development opportunities for your direct reports. The same philosophy holds true for your own professional development. What is your PIE in the Sky? What gets your juices going at work? What would you like to do more of, and how can you create opportunities for your own intellectual advancement?

This advancement can take place through a variety of formal or informal actions. Creative problem-solving, innovation exercises, and team building are all vehicles for self-development. The goal is finding activities that are not adding stress to your workday but decreasing stress. Partnering with staff or other managers works well.

Start a Book Group

A great way to stimulate your brain is to create a book club at work. Gather a group of your peers (nurse managers or other managers in your organization) and pick a book to read. The topics could be management related, health care related, or just plain fun. Set up lunch meetings and meet in the cafeteria or use a conference room and brown bag it. Take turns with other people to lead the discussion at each gathering.

To get you started, here are questions that work for any book:

- What parts of the book resonate with you and why?
- What will you think or do differently as a result of reading the book?
- What questions would you ask the author if you could?
- What bothered you about the book?
- What other thoughts do you have?

You might start with a quarterly meeting to allow everyone plenty of time to read the book. Let the club make recommendations for future books. Start with this book.

Time-Saver Tools
Book Group Guide

I've expanded on the questions listed above to make your first Book Group meeting pain free and easy to plan for as you discuss this book.

www.HiringFiringInspiring.com

Oliver Wendell Holmes Jr. wisely said, "A mind once stretched by a new idea never regains its original dimension." Because of this phenomenon, engaging in professional development provides short-term and long-term results. Short term, you are energized and get better outcomes through your new learning or viewpoints. Long term, you grow and develop and avoid the trap of being in a rut.

As a newer manager, you have the responsibility to continue the development of your management skills. Your boss and your direct reports will appreciate your efforts while they watch you grow and mature in your leadership role. It might sound cliché, but take it one step at a time and enjoy the journey.

Working with Your Boss

Having a positive, collaborative relationship with your manager provides the foundation for your relationships with your direct reports. If your relationship is strained or dysfunctional, then your overall job will be more difficult, and the staff who report to you will feel the effects of this stress. When you are comfortable and feel supported, it's much easier to effectively manage your direct reports because you have a positive role model and a system to follow.

We all come to work with preconceived beliefs and mindsets about bosses; the first step is to clearly identify your presumptions. By looking at deep-seated ideas, you gain insight into the voices you hear when it comes to your connection with your manager. For example, one nurse manager said, "I've never had a boss who was onsite. I figured 'no news was good news,' so when Mark [her manager] kept showing up to check in, I took it personally. I thought he was questioning my abilities. I came to find that he does this with everyone. That's just his style. Now I appreciate him dropping by, and it makes it easy for us to stay in touch. The staff also likes that he knows what's going on in our department." Knowing what your beliefs are can help you work more effectively with your boss.

Beliefs and Mind-sets about Bosses

Take a few minutes to answer these questions:

- What beliefs and mind-sets about bosses did you learn growing up? (Think about those dinner conversations you heard.)
- What beliefs and mind-sets about supervisor/direct report relationships have you learned since you started working? (Think about your past bosses and their bosses.)
- What effect do these beliefs have on your current relationship with your boss?

This exercise is also great to do with other managers so that you can create a dialogue and explore how these beliefs and mind-sets might be helping or hurting how you and your boss work together.

Creating positive connections with your boss results in a variety of benefits, including the following:

- Decreased stress
- Increased visibility
- Opportunities for growth
- Stronger connection to the organization overall
- Potential for learning more

Unfortunately, obstacles often get in the way of creating these positive connections. They may include your work beliefs, personality conflicts, being too passive, a boss who is never around or a know-it-all, or a no news is good news philosophy. If you take the time to identify the obstacles, you can put in the work it takes to forge a positive connection.

Get to Know Your Boss

One way to build on your relationship with your supervisor is to better understand what his or her job is like. Here are helpful questions to ask to learn more:

- What is your PIE in the Sky?
- What's keeping you up at night?
- What are the nagging worries that you face that I can positively impact?
- Where do you spend most of your time at work?
- What else do I need to know about your job?

Try asking these questions in a one-on-one meeting and see where the dialogue goes. If you'd like, ask to attend an executive team meeting as an observer or go along to meetings outside the organization. Learn what it's like to be in his or her shoes and you'll be better positioned to support your boss, department, and the organization.

If you want to be an effective, inspiring nurse manager, you need to forge a positive relationship with your boss. It's nearly impossible to navigate the twists and turns of most workplaces today without support from your direct supervisor. You need him or her to run interference for you, gain access to information that you don't have, and help you understand the nuances of the organization. Most managers are happy to help. Stephen Covey wisely said, "Seek first to understand, then be understood." When it comes to bosses, learn first, and then share your thoughts, and you'll always get better results.

Finding a Mentor

When we talk about mentors at work, the idea of a trusted colleague who has more experience comes to mind. The mentor knows how to do the job of the mentee. She or he has been where the mentee is and understands the challenges to being successful in the role. The mentor knows the organizational landscape and helps the mentee find her or his way around political landmines and avoid organizational quicksand. The mentor also joins in the celebration of success and forward progress.

Because my focus here is taking care of yourself, you want to find a mentor who is wise, willing to teach, and acts as a supporter. The mentor should help you solve problems, brainstorm innovative ideas, and find ways to cope with your day-to-day challenges. Several nurse managers in my focus groups commented on the value of having a mentor within the organization. They pointed out that the mentor is not your boss, but instead someone who is a peer with experience and knowledge to share.

Mentor Search

Looking for a mentor and not sure where to start? Usually, the selection process is "organic"—it just seems to happen as you meet with people and get to know them. If you want to make the process more formal, the guidelines from the Society for Human Resource Management (2009) state that a successful mentor should have the following qualifications:

- Willingness to assume and visibly demonstrate leadership.
- Demonstrated people-oriented behavior.
- Regarded as successful in the organization.
- Knowledge of the company's vision, mission, goals, culture, policies, and programs.
- Commitment to developing staff.
- Willingness to share personal experiences relevant to the goals of the protégé.
- Willingness to develop goals, to coach, and to give feedback.

Keep these factors in mind while you move ahead in the mentor-selection process.

Finding a mentor helps both you and the mentor. The person doing the teaching strengthens his or her leadership skills and knowledge and feels good about helping someone else grow and develop. You, the protégé, benefit from getting a perspective from someone who has more experience. Trust is the hallmark of a great protégé/ mentor relationship. Confidentiality is imperative so that you can ask "dumb" questions and the mentor can share candid responses.

Most people find that a strong mentoring relationship is life changing in the support that it offers for both parties. After you have a feel for what mentoring is all about, you might want to start mentoring someone. "Paying it forward" is one of the best ways to thank your mentor.

Summary

Taking care of yourself is an underlying element of the Partnership Protocol model for inspiring managers. A complimentary focus on life outside of work is critical because it provides you the equilibrium you need to do everything else. Finding time for professional development and growth opportunities is another way to take care of yourself. For example, teaching—or becoming a student again— can provide you an avenue for development. You can also decrease stress and enhance your job satisfaction by creating and maintaining positive connections with your boss Finally, finding a mentor is another way of taking care of yourself. When employees are making you crazy, your boss is frustrating you, and the world seems to be falling down around you, your mentor is there to listen, offer support, and help you figure out a way to move forward.

Don't think you are being selfish when you put on your own oxygen mask first. Instead, think about how inspired you are and, as a result, how inspiring you can be to others.

PART III
Resignations and Firings

We've spent the bulk of this book talking about making wise hiring decisions and tactical steps for inspiring yourself and others. Now the stakes are even higher as you face the possibility of losing a valued team member or asking a poor performer to go. Either way, proven steps for minimizing the pain and maximizing the gain will guide you in these interactions..

In this part of the book, I guide you through the process of voluntary resignations—those that are initiated by the employee. Chapter 14 includes how to conduct a useful exit interview, track data, and stay in touch. Chapter 15 focuses on effective practices for performance management, including managing someone out of the organization (the firing process). Additionally, I walk you through the necessary steps to let someone go, with due process and a focus on respect and dignity.

Please note that this part is designed to provide general information on a variety of employment issues that may arise, but does not address the specific requirements of federal, state, or local laws. Please consult with your HR department or legal counsel with questions and to ensure compliance.

CHAPTER 14
Voluntary Resignations

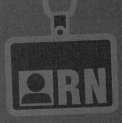

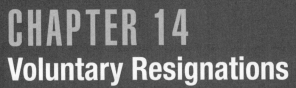

Voluntary separations are usually disappointing. Presumably, you've been working hard to manage and motivate this staff member, and now he or she is leaving. You will have one of two reactions.

- "Yes! This will save me the hassle of having to fire this person."
- "Oh no! I'm sorry that he or she is leaving."

Either way, visions of the hiring process and its ensuing work start to enter into your mind. You worry about how others will take the news. Will the employee who is leaving be taking other folks along to his or her new job? How will you cover the vacancy in your staffing?

Accepting the Resignation

Before you go too far down the "How is this is going to affect me?" path, focus on the employee who has just resigned. If you want the person to stay, try the following conversation pointers:

- Congratulate the employee on his or her new job.
- Ask where he or she is going and what the job entails.
- If appropriate, ask whether you can do anything to get him or her to stay.

Employees leave organizations for all kinds of reasons—both personal and professional. If the resignation stems from personal changes, such as relocation, you have little chance of that person staying. If the resignation stems from a change in lifestyle, such as staying home with aging parents or children or going back to school, discuss more flexible scheduling or part-time work. If this is a top performer, get creative and see whether you can find a compromise that might work.

If the employee is leaving because he or she is pursuing different career choices (such as a change in clinical specialty), or a different work environment (such as a move from a hospital setting to a clinic), you might not be able to come up with a viable alternative. Listen for the real reason someone is leaving. According to James K. Harter, PhD (2008), Gallup's chief scientist for workplace management, "At least 75% of the reasons for voluntary turnover can be influenced by managers." Most of these reasons directly relate to the effective execution of the Partnership Protocol. If you need reminders, revisit Part II, "Inspiring."

Next Steps

Arrrgh (to quote a famous pirate)—resignations stink! To make the best of it, focus on what is within your control. How can you manage the process so that this employee leaves with a good feeling about you, your department, and the organization? If the employee is definitely leaving, here are a few suggestions to help the process run smoothly:

- If you haven't received a written letter of resignation, ask the employee to write one.

- Refer to your organization's policy manual or work with HR to ensure all separation procedures are addressed, including the employee's rights and benefits such as last pay date, sick leave, vacation pay out, and so on

- Notify other staff members that the employee is leaving— talk with the employee who has resigned about how the notification will happen.

- Agree upon the final day of work. Start the process of transitioning work duties if applicable. Facilitate cross-training of responsibilities to other staff members immediately to avoid gaps in service delivery.

- If you are okay with the employee giving notice and don't necessarily want to push him or her to stay, start the process of filling the position as soon as possible by posting the job internally and on job boards. This avoids any problems if the employee attempts to rescind his or her resignation later because you are already actively trying to fill the position.

- Ask the employee to update his or her job description so that when you start the Hiring SMARTT process (covered in Part I of this book) you are one step ahead in the game.

- Schedule an exit interview with a third party—usually HR or your manager—to get feedback from the employee. This is very helpful in spotting trends regarding the reasons that employees leave your department.

- If this employee is someone you would gladly rehire, let the employee know that you would like to keep in touch periodically. Make a note to send a holiday or birthday card, or invite him or her to department gatherings.

Time-Saver Tools

Resignation Checklist

Print out these reminders so you don't miss anything important when an employee leaves.

www.HiringFiringInspiring.com

What can you learn from this resignation? What retention strategies bubble up from conversations with employees who are leaving? The "only if …" sentiments that you hear should raise a red flag for actions you might be able to take to prevent others from leaving.

The idea here is to keep the door open for future employment. You want employees to leave with a good feeling about your organization so that they talk about their time working with you in positive terms. Many nurse managers report that employees leave looking for greener pastures and quickly realize that they had it pretty good. If you keep the door open, your turnover costs decrease significantly because of the quick ramp up to full productivity when you rehire a top-performing employee.

The Boomerang Program

Jason Nemoy, PHR, (personal communication, 2009), former senior manager of recruiting for California Pizza Kitchen, Inc. (CPK) shared their "Boomerang" program for rehiring top-performing employees. CPK recruiters and managers stayed in touch with former employees via letters, newsletters, and quick notes. "This created an ongoing connection, and 8-10% of people who left came back." They also asked the people who left on good terms to refer others they thought would fit the culture well. The efforts paid off and valuable former employees returned.

Summary

When voluntary resignations occur, sometimes you're relieved and other times you're sad. The best you can do when someone leaves is to part on good terms. Be aware that employees who remain will be watching you to see how you respond and how quickly the team rebounds. Also, use this time to learn. The resignation gives you a chance to look at assignments with fresh eyes and to make changes based on feedback from the exit interview.

Goodbyes are a difficult part of management life, so use your support mechanisms to get back on track and put the focus on the people who are working with you. They will appreciate it, and so will your customers.

CHAPTER 15
Involuntary Terminations

Voluntary Resignations

Involuntary Terminations

The following statements are survey quotes from nurse managers who responded to the question "What is your biggest challenge when it comes to terminating employees?"

- "I feel guilty that I could have done more to help the employee be more successful."
- "It is the part of my job that I hate the most."
- "I personally don't like to make mistakes, so I will put off the inevitable so I can make sure my decision is right."

You have probably experienced similar feelings in your role as a manager, and I'm sure you can empathize with these managers. Firing employees is difficult; however, being knowledgeable and prepared helps the process go more smoothly. As I focus on involuntary separation of employees in this chapter, I share specific strategies for the following:

- Managing performance as a foundation for any termination.
- Administering the discipline process.
- Having the termination conversation.
- Managing grievances and going to court.

The focus in this chapter is for-cause separations, when employee actions have led to the termination. As uncomfortable as terminating an employee is, the payoff is typically worth the effort. Most employees who are terminated involuntarily are repeatedly guilty of at least one of the following transgressions:

- Underperforming on the job.
- Spreading negative attitudes.
- Making costly mistakes.
- Not coming to work on time (or at all).

When you let employees get away with these behaviors, you are sending a message to your customers and other staff members—and it's not a positive one. The message to staff is that failing to meet the stated expectations for your area is okay and that you have different standards for different people. You also inadvertently let your customers know the service your area provides is inconsistent at best and poor at worst. I'm betting these are not the messages you want to convey as the leader in your department.

Not convinced yet? I know some managers think that *any* body is better than *no* body, but I disagree. Employees who demonstrate negative behaviors are costing you, your department, and the organization time, energy, money, and your area's reputation. Experienced managers share that once a poor performer is terminated, they hear things like this:

- Our team works well together now that _____ is gone.
- The feeling around here is much more positive now that _____ is gone.
- I didn't realize how much of _____'s work I was doing.
- I'm glad _____ is gone and that we've reallocated her duties.
- Thank you for taking a stand on _____ being late all the time.

In my survey, nurses said they wished their nurse manager would start

- Upholding unit standards and disciplining those who aren't meeting the standards.
- Firing people who are chronically late.
- Holding people accountable for their actions.
- Addressing staff and physician behavior issues that decrease morale and potentially affect patient care negatively.

The staff is counting on you to be a strong and consistent leader, and one aspect of that is to manage the effects of others' poor behavior.

A small group of people may defend the actions of the terminated employee and portray you as the bad guy. They typically do this out of misguided loyalty and maybe fear—especially if they are demonstrating some of the same negative behaviors as the employee who was let go. You can address their concerns one on one; just be sure to hold all staff accountable consistently and fairly, as covered in Part II. When employees know what to expect from you regarding their performance, they're more likely to support your decisions.

> ### Keep Staff Informed
>
> After an employee is terminated, hold a meeting or send an e-mail to let staff know that the person is gone. This helps dispel rumors. Of course, you can't share private matters with staff members, but you can say something like, "I want to let you know that Bobby has left the organization as of today. Of course, I can't share the details of what happened because they are private. If you have any questions or concerns, please come and see me."
>
> Share plans for hiring, recognize those who have been doing a good job, and talk with staff members who are directly involved about their ideas for sharing work responsibilities until someone else is hired. If appropriate, ask them for input on temporarily reorganizing how the work is done. Avoid the temptation to make decisions entirely on your own because this decreases buy-in from others in the department. This is the time to use your skills to foster open communication.
>
> Your open-door policy will come in handy if employees want to discuss the separation with you or have questions. Letting staff know when a team member leaves fosters open communication, creates and builds relationships, and supports team members. These elements of the Partnership Protocol are important when terminating an employee involuntarily because you want remaining employees to continue the work at hand.

Performance Management

The key to effectively terminating an employee is comprehensive performance management. The words are performance + management, not performance ignoring or performance micromanaging. As we have discussed throughout Part II of this book, your role is to create an environment where employees can be successful. When you consistently and fairly share information (the *what*, the *why*, and the *how* from the Performance Platform) and provide feedback (informally and formally), you are providing employees with the tools they need to succeed.

If involuntary separation of the employee is likely, then either the initial hiring decision was incorrect or the employee has decided not to (or is unable to) continue his or her commitment to doing the work as assigned. Either way, you can only control what is on your side of the performance management equation. In a survey, I asked, "What is your biggest challenge when it comes to firing?" One nurse manager wisely answered, "I have none, especially when it is related to poor practice." Keep this confident approach in mind while you tackle the process of terminating an employee.

The Boiling Frog

Have you heard the story of the boiling frog? This story says that if you put a frog in cold water and slowly turn up the heat, he will die because he doesn't feel the subtle changes in the water temperature. Conversely, if you place the frog in boiling water, he will jump out because he knows the water is too hot to survive.

The point of this story is that we often fail to notice as changes happen over time. This relates to involuntary terminations of employees because in many cases managers do not see the trend that is occurring with employee performance problems. The performance issues happen gradually and everyone gets used to the poor results. The slow rise in temperature (poor performance) is ignored and the co-workers and patients are the ones who feel the effects. On the other hand, if an employee comes to work and has one egregious behavior problem (such as yelling at a patient), the manager notices and the employee is terminated. The morale of the story is to pay attention to poor performers and take action early and often.

Please remember that the goal of performance management is an employee who demonstrates the desired behaviors for his or her job consistently and successfully. Janet Ladd, SPHR, (personal communication, 2009) HR professional with more than 20 years of experience, said this: "Remember that the goal of performance management is to create alignment between the organization's goals and individual contributions toward the achievement of the goals. Ideally, it aligns people's passions and talents with the needs of the organization." This conforms with what we discussed about performance management in the beginning of Part II.

When looking at individual performance, you want to focus on the elements that impact the employee performing the job successfully:

- **Ability:** If you notice performance gaps, the first element to look at is ability. Ask yourself whether the employee has the knowledge, skills, and aptitude to do the work. Have you provided the *how* for the performance, including education and training? Can the employee demonstrate competency when asked? You need to know whether the person has the ability to succeed.

- **Opportunity:** You've heard the saying practice makes perfect. Sometimes staff members aren't proficient with workplace behaviors because they don't have the opportunity to perform the task often enough. In this case, provide policies and procedures that employees can refer to regarding work performed infrequently. When performance is sagging because of a lack of opportunity to perform the task, learning aides (such as a card with steps on it) can help to solve the problem.

- **Motivation:** Does the employee have an internal desire or passion for doing the work? Is he or she engaged in performing work duties because of internal motivators or does he or she need pushing from an outside source? Motivation is a crucial element of effective performance; as the old saying goes, "You can lead a horse to water, but you cannot make him drink."

Ability and opportunity are easier elements to correct. If a lack of ability or opportunity is the cause of the problem and the staff member is motivated to improve, then coaching, feedback, and learning aids usually help move the performance toward the desired goal of competent execution. Unfortunately, a lack of motivation is much harder to influence and is more often the cause of poor performance. If you need help with improving an employee's motivation, revisit the five components of the Partnership Protocol in Part II; after all, they are the foundation for improving employee engagement and ultimately performance.

While you use the Performance Platform (see Part II of this book) to elevate performance, notice early whether the deficiency stems from a lack of ability, opportunity, or motivation so that your solution is appropriately implemented. Make sure you are clear when sharing the *what,* the *why*, and the *how* and that your feedback is consistent and fair. Noticing gaps in performance early saves you time in the long run, and performance management lays the groundwork for involuntary separation if the employee repeatedly fails to meet or exceed the required performance levels.

Working with Human Resources

I've stated many times throughout this book that your partnership with HR is important to your success as a manager. When hiring, you benefit from HR's assistance and input on your selection choices. When inspiring, HR can provide support for your initiatives through growth and development or coaching and feedback. When it comes to termination, HR provides expert guidance on how to effectively dismiss someone and minimize the legal risk of doing so. If you don't have an HR resource, ask for help from your boss, an experienced management peer, or the organization's legal counsel. Do not try to terminate an employee without support from someone who is knowledgeable about the proper procedures—you don't need to go through this alone.

Unfortunately, almost half of the 53 nurse manager respondents to my survey question "What's your biggest challenge when it comes to terminating employees?" included human resources and/or the complexity of the documentation. I believe that these two challenges are directly connected. Of the following responses, what do you notice if you take out the emotion and read between the lines?

- "Human resources slowdown."

- "HR and having to be consistent in an organization where the documentation of work behavior issues were there but nothing was ever done about it."

- "Having documented every single infraction along the way in such a way that HR feels it is enough. HR reps all saying the same thing."

- "The obstacles that HR sets up, still making you go through the motions of the dreaded Performance Improvement Plan when you know in your gut that the employee is not going to cut it. It just prolongs the agony."

I'm not trying to take sides here, but do you see the themes? The comments really demonstrate the need for due process before termination (that is, a process based on established rules and procedures that are both fair and consistently applied). When you read the challenges objectively, you can see why the policies and procedures exist and why HR sometimes slows down the process to make sure all the Is are dotted and the Ts are crossed. What nurse managers often realize when they approach involuntary separation is that they should have gone to HR earlier in the coaching process. The employee doesn't meet expectations repeatedly but the manager sees each infraction as minor and looks the other way until finally reaching his or her boiling point—at which point HR says, "Slow down." The manager has had months to think about all the infractions, but the employee (and HR) is just hearing about it and steps are missing from the process. Without following the outlined organizational policies and procedures and having an objective attention to detail, the organization is exposed to unnecessary legal risks and financial hardship.

Working with Unions

Contrary to popular belief, when working with union employees, the job of termination may just be easier because the contract spells out very clearly the due process for terminating an employee. That is if you know the contract. Barbara Bartels (personal communication, 2009), a senior HR business partner with a large community hospital and many years of experience terminating union employees, says, "As a manager, it's in your best interest to review and understand the management rights that are included in the contract. Since the steps for responding to discipline are usually clearly spelled out, you have better success with the process if you know it inside and out."

She goes on to say, "Don't rely on so called staff experts or union reps who say they know the contract—make sure you know it yourself. It's also a great idea to talk with your HR representative to learn more about the union agreement and the discipline process. He or she can be very helpful in translating the information for you."

A union contract ends up being the bad cop when you are going through the progressive discipline process. You can quote the management rights when working with a staff member. For example, "We are meeting today to talk about your lateness to work. This is your fifth occurrence. Your union contract clearly states that after five episodes of tardiness, I must issue a written discipline regardless of the circumstances. Here is the written warning that states that if you are late again, you will be issued a final warning and ultimately if the pattern continues, you will be fired. Do you understand what I have just reviewed with you or do you have any questions?"

Know the contract and your rights as a manager, and then you are in a stronger position for terminating underperforming union employees.

Getting to know your HR generalist or business partner is vital to your ability to coach employees to termination or promotion. HR professionals understand employee relations and the legal implications of your coaching behaviors. The more you know, the better prepared you are to minimize the ramifications of terminating an employee.

The Discipline Process

According to S. Heathfield (2009), "Progressive discipline is a process for dealing with job-related behavior that does not meet expected and communicated performance standards. The primary purpose for progressive discipline is to assist the employee to understand that a performance problem or opportunity for improvement exists." I like this definition because it is developmental—it focuses on helping the employee solve the problem. Progressive discipline should never feel like a witch hunt or persecution, and as the manager, you play a major role in the perceptions that exist around discipline.

Notice how the definition says "does not meet expected and communicated performance standards." Sound familiar? Think about the legs of the Performance Platform discussed in Part II. Sharing the *what,* the *why,* and the *how* with employees early lays a foundation for their strong performance and for the progressive discipline process. Also note the primary purpose is to "assist the employee to understand." That's where informal and formal feedback come into play. Without these elements in place, the Performance Platform falls flat and so does the employee.

The progressive discipline process varies from organization to organization, but there are usually common components. Your policy and procedure manual, manager, HR representative, and legal counsel are all excellent resources for you to learn more about the process to follow. You'll want to know the policies so that you aren't blindsided by unexpected steps that require you to go back to the beginning of the process.

The Society for Human Resource Management (SHRM) shares five principles for effective discipline (2008). To be effective, discipline needs to be:

- **Corrective:** Attempts to improve performance.
- **Fair:** Free from bias.
- **Consistent:** Delivered uniformly.
- **Progressive:** One step builds on the next.
- **Due process:** Based on established rules.

Each of the ideas offers a good rule of thumb for busy managers. Before you embark on the disciplinary process, make sure you consider these important principles.

Most progressive discipline policies include the following steps for at-will employees. According to Lawyers.com, "An employee is employed at the will of the employer for as little or as long as the private employer wishes, and in whatever lawful capacity the employer requires. The employee may choose to work at the employee's will for the length of time he or she desires. An employer need not provide any reason for terminating an 'at will' employee, so long as the termination isn't unlawful or discriminatory (based on age, sex, national origin, disability)." Although you have the right to terminate employees at will, conventional wisdom suggests that a well-thought-out process is more constructive and leads to better results for everyone involved. Your organization's policy or HR staff will define the timing for using these steps and give guidelines to follow for periods of time between infractions so that you know when to start from the beginning again.

With this in mind, the formal progressive discipline steps in many organizations for nonunion employees are as follows:

1. Verbal warning
2. Written warning
3. Final warning (with or without suspension)
4. Termination

Please keep in mind that these steps begin after the elements of the Performance Platform have been exercised. You have clearly shared the *what,* the *why*, and the *how* of behaviors with the employee and have provided feedback on their performance up to this point. The behavior and performance are not meeting the agreed upon standards; hence, the progressive discipline process.

What Do I Say?

Managers are often unsure what to say during each of the steps of the discipline process. Here are ideas for what to say at each stage leading up to termination. Of course, you'll want to practice with another manager until you feel comfortable with what to say. You'll also want to add your own style to the conversation to be as genuine as possible.

continues

- **Verbal warning:** "Sam, this is the third time I've talked to you about being away from the reception desk for long periods of time. We've talked about why it's important for you to be there for our patients and strategies for getting your work done or getting coverage when you do need to leave. According to our progressive discipline process, this is a verbal warning to let you know how serious this is. I need for you to stay at the desk when the clinic is open. Of course, you need to take your two breaks and lunch, and you can ask Sarah to cover you when you leave. Otherwise, if you need to take care of a work-related project that requires you to be away from the desk, talk to the charge nurse or me before you go anywhere. Do you have any questions? Do you understand how important this is? I'll be following up with an e-mail to confirm what I've just said for your records and mine. If this happens again, I will issue a written warning, but I hope that doesn't happen. Thanks, and I'm counting on you to be there for the patients."

- **Written warning:** "Sam, I was in the clinic today looking for you and couldn't find you anywhere. Lydia (the charge nurse) said she did not know where you were. What happened? (Listen to his response.) I understand that you had to go and pick up the report from the lab because the fax is broken, but I asked you to let me or the charge nurse know if you were leaving. I didn't know and neither did Lydia.

  — As I told you in our last meeting, if this happened again, then I would be issuing a written warning. I wanted to hear what you had to say so that I could include your comments. As you know from our last conversation, this is very serious. Do you understand why it's so important for you to be here when the clinic is open? According to the discipline process, the next step, if you are missing in action again, is a final warning (with suspension if applicable). Please stay on the unit so that doesn't happen. I'll type up the written warning and include what you told me today. I'll have it for you tomorrow to sign with a copy for you and for me."

- **Final warning:** "Sam, I'm very disappointed that we are having this conversation again. I was in the clinic today and you were no where to be found and the desk was empty. I asked Sarah and Lydia where you were and neither of them knew. It seems like the job working at the reception desk isn't suiting you well. Sam, this is your final warning. If you are not at the desk or on an approved break or business related outing with prior permission, then you will be terminated. Do you understand? Please sign this final warning, and here is your copy."

You can see that most of what you are saying at each juncture is simply what you observed or was reported to you and the consequences of those actions. Be direct, factual, and prepared. You can empathize with the employee, but remember the standards and expectations for all employees and stand your ground—even if the employee argues, cries, or shuts down. Ask someone from HR to join you if you are worried about the employee's response and for corroboration of the conversation. Always follow up in writing.

The "Hot Stove" Rule

In a question-and-answer e-mail with HR professionals at the Society for Human Resource Management (SHRM), one consultant shared this advice comparing the disciplinary process to touching a hot stove: Discipline, just as the result of touching a hot stove, must follow a warning and must be immediate, consistent, and impersonal.

Following the rule, disciplinary action must

- Occur after a warning has been ignored (just as a burn occurs from ignoring the warning a hot stove gives).

- Occur immediately (just as a hot stove burns immediately).

- Be consistent (just as a hot stove burns every time).

- Be impersonal in that it occurs regardless of who the person is (just as a hot stove burns any and every person who touches it) (2008).

The progressive discipline process is in place to help both you and the employee by keeping communication out in the open. Strive for transparency in your dealings with employees who are demonstrating performance problems. Be upfront about the *what,* the *why*, and the *how* and provide clear, consistent feedback to ensure that you are doing everything you possibly can to help the employee succeed. If I sound like a broken record here, then note the importance of following these steps to decrease your frustration and increase your effectiveness as a manager.

The Termination Meeting

You've done everything you can to keep the employee onboard. You've used the Partnership Protocol, the Performance Platform, and had multiple conversations without a change in performance. You've moved through the stages of the progressive discipline process and issued a final warning. The employee has demonstrated the problem behavior again, and it's time for the termination.

First, you want to meet with HR or the organization's legal counsel to make sure that you have done everything possible to work with this employee. I know it might not seem fair that the burden of proof is on your shoulders, but unfortunately, that's the way it works. Here is a termination checklist with key questions to discuss in this meeting.

Termination Checklist

- Who from HR will be present during the termination meeting? It's always better to have two people present.

- Are all documents prepared that need to be signed or given to the employee? (COBRA, final paycheck, vacation payout, and so on)

- Who will collect the employee's name badge, pager, locker key, and such?

- How will you handle the employee packing his or her personal belongings? Do you need to have a box ready? Will the person have the option to come back another time to pick things up to avoid embarrassment?

- Have you notified security to be on call in case you need assistance?

- Do you need to change computer passwords or disconnect from shared drives before you have your meeting so that the employee can't tamper with records?

- Who will check the employee's belongings when he or she leaves? (This is to protect the employee and the organization.)

- Who should the employee contact if he or she has questions in the future?

- Is there anything else you are forgetting?

Time-Saver Tools
Termination Meeting Checklist

Having to fire an employee is an emotional event. Use this check-list to stay on track.

www.HiringFiringInspiring.com

When you have the answers to all these questions, you are ready for the conversation. There are different schools of thought on the best time of day and day of the week for letting someone go. Those you fire on a Friday afternoon have all weekend to stew about it without any way to move forward. Conversely, if you terminate employees earlier in the week, usually at the end of the day, you provide them with an opportunity to take care of any unfinished business, start making plans to look for a new job, and so on. If you ask someone to leave at the beginning of his or her shift, you'll have a gap in staffing that may prove difficult to fill.

In *101 Tough Conversations to Have with Employees*, Paul Fal-cone (2009) shares this script for beginning the conversation when terminating for cause:

> *I'm calling this meeting to let you know that I'm afraid we're going to have to separate your employment today. As you know, we've been going through a number of interventions with you regarding your overall performance on the job, both via verbal and written notices, and I'm afraid that we've made the decision to go our separate ways.*

The script goes on to cover what happens next, the procedure for leaving the building, and so on. If you are uncomfortable with hav-ing tough conversations, the book is a great resource for many situ-ations, including termination.

Practice Makes Perfect

Before you hold a termination conversation, practice what you will say with someone from HR or another manager. Have the person who is helping you act out the following tough situations so that you'll be more comfortable handling them:

- "I'm not signing anything, and you can't make me!"
- "I didn't do anything wrong—you are just singling me out because I'm _____."
- "You're not being fair; you let (someone else) do the same thing and didn't fire her."
- "I didn't mean to, I'm really sorry, I can't lose my job… (breaks into tears)."
- "You've got a lot of nerve. If you did your job better, we wouldn't be here. I'd like to fire you for being a bad manager…."

You'll find that practicing these tough situations in advance will greatly increase your comfort level during the actual meeting. You might even be pleasantly surprised when the employee says, "You're right; this isn't the job for me."

The feedback I received from nurse manager focus groups was to make the termination conversation "short and sweet"—no apologies, no long stories or confusing messages with compliments to make you feel better. The consensus seemed to be that terminating an employee will always be difficult, and if you get to the point where it isn't, then maybe it's time for you to stop managing.

Grievances and Going to Court

Even when you follow all the outlined steps for the progressive discipline process, employees will act surprised that they are being fired. They might accuse you of unfair treatment or a lack of understanding. They might cry, argue, or storm out of the room. Be prepared for any type of response and have support available nearby. When an employee feels disgruntled about being terminated, he or she might file for unemployment or seek an attorney for a possible lawsuit. This is why having HR involved and completing all the requisite paperwork is so important. If you are called into an unemployment hearing, you want to have all your ducks in a row so that you can defend your position.

States create their own unemployment laws, and overarching federal laws apply as well. Because your job is to manage a patient care unit, you do not need to become a legal expert in these matters. Use your resources. During the termination process, if you think the employee might create claims of discrimination, let HR and your legal counsel know right away. You know this employee; you've been working with him or her and have seen reactions to other situations. Do you think he or she will fight you on this? If so, be prepared. In all cases, make sure you have adequate documentation to defend your decision to terminate this employee (for example, job descriptions, signed employee handbooks, copies of e-mails, documentation of oral warnings, copies of written warnings).

If an employee does file for unemployment benefits, your organization can choose to pay them or fight the payment. HR staff are trained to determine which option makes more sense. They might even use a third-party administrator to work with unemployment claims. According to Shawn Smith and Rebecca Mazin, in their *HR Answer Book* (2004), "Most states do not allow employees fired for serious cause or misconduct to collect benefits." They go on to say, "Merely having a difficult personality, being a sloppy worker, or not being skilled enough to perform a job are not sufficient justification to deny someone unemployment benefits." According to the Maryland Department of Labor, Licensing, and Regulation, "Unemployment insurance is an employer funded insurance program which provides benefits to persons who are unemployed through no fault of their own and who are ready, willing, and able to work." This is standard language found in most unemployment insurance statutes, and as you can immediately see, the phrase "through no fault of their own" leaves a lot of unanswered questions. Obviously, there are many gray areas when it comes to unemployment benefits, so I'll say it again: Ask for help.

If you contest the payment of benefits, you will be asked to appear at the claims office for a hearing. Bring all your documentation. Bring job descriptions, signed employee handbooks, copies of emails, documentation of oral warnings, copies of written warnings, and so on. You might be asked to bring paperwork from other terminations to prove you have treated this employee consistently with others. You won't wonder why HR is so insistent on complete paperwork after your first visit to a claims hearing to defend a termination. Most likely, you'll be grateful for how prepared you feel.

Finally, if you are sued for wrongful termination, you will be working with an attorney who will walk you through the proceedings and direct you through the next steps. I hope this will be a rare occurrence. And, although you cannot control whether someone sues you, you can control how prepared you are and how you respond. If you have consistently and fairly used the Performance Platform for managing behavior, and you have followed your organization's progressive discipline policies (including appropriate documentation), you will be ready to defend your position in court. This is a last resort, and I hope you will never have to experience it.

Summary

Involuntary separations are never a pleasant experience. Even when warranted, the process is stressful because we all understand the magnitude of losing a job. As an effective manager, and to minimize the pain, you want to pay careful attention to these areas:

- Execute consistent strategies for effective performance management as a foundation for any for-cause separation.
- Work closely with HR.
- Consistently administer the discipline process.
- Practice the termination conversation.
- Be prepared for grievances and going to court.

This is a part of your job that you want to avoid, and you can do so by hiring the right person for the right job and managing performance (both positive and negative) consistently and routinely. Even when you do everything right, however, it takes two to tango, and each employee must decide to come to work, ready to work. When it doesn't work out, do what you know is right for all and let the person go. In the end, you'll be glad you did (and most of the time, so will he or she).

EPILOGUE

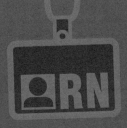

Congratulations on finishing the book. This is your chance to recharge, refocus, and recommit to the powerfully important role you hold as a nurse manager. Now is the time to look at the hiring, firing, and inspiring parts of your job from a big-picture perspective.

When it comes to hiring, your responsibility is to find the person who fits your department by Hiring SMARTT. That means thoughtfully looking at the open job and the desired strengths. Then you progress to making a list of relevant behavior-based questions for each interview. You ask the questions and listen carefully to the responses, you review the responses, and you take the time to make a well informed decision. Most managers stop here, but as a Hiring SMARTT manager, you know that thoughtfully bringing the person onboard is a key differentiator in engaging the employee from the first day.

Next, we looked at what it means to be an inspiring nurse manager. Are you feeling inspired? Using the Partnership Protocol as a guide, you have a framework that starts with aligning your actions with the vision and values of the organization and your department. Fostering open communication, creating and building relationships, and supporting team members are at the core of being an inspiring manager. One last element of engaging employees is encouraging growth and development. Use the Performance Platform to have regular coaching conversations with staff to stay on track with engagement and performance.

Finally, we looked at the tough times that can result from resignations and involuntary terminations. Don't worry; you will be prepared for these tough times if you use the tools and techniques shared by many wise nurse managers and HR professionals with years of experience. Just take it one step at a time and ask for help along the way.

As our time together comes to an end, imagine for a moment that you are in a hovercraft floating above yourself at work on a typical day. You are an objective observer watching all your moves from arrival to departure. How are you doing? What do you see? Hear? Think? Feel?

Sometimes we get so wrapped up in the "doing" that we lose sight of the "being." Not to get too esoteric, but take a few minutes now to stop reading, sit still, and contemplate your role as a nurse manager. Allow yourself the freedom to answer the following questions in a thoughtful, objective, hovercraft-like manner.

- Who have I brought to our team that's a great fit and how has he or she contributed to our department's results?

- What transformational ideas have I introduced that helped my staff feel more engaged at work?

- In what ways have the patients that we serve healed as a result of our work with them?

I hope you can let yourself experience the satisfaction and joy of making a difference. We have all had experiences that have been challenging and we have come out on the other side with a new sense of clarity and appreciation (most of the time, anyway).

By hiring the right people who fit in your department, inspiring those who are there, and saying goodbye to those who need to go, you have the opportunity to make a positive difference in the lives of many people every day. Not everyone can honestly say that.

APPENDIX
Time-Saver Tools

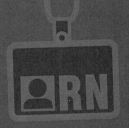

I want to save you time on your hiring, firing and inspiring journey so I've created these take-away tools to make your life easier. Need a form? Not sure about an agenda for a staff meeting? Check www.HiringFiringInspiring.com first.

The tools are listed by chapter to make the reference point easier to find. Now is not the time to reinvent the wheel—just utilize these as my gift and use the time you save to go hang out with the staff. Enjoy!

Chapter 1

A+ Candidate Strengths Inventory

Chapter 2

Behavior Based Questions Prep Form

Chapter 3

Interview Notes

Share Day Feedback Form

Chapter 5

Applicant Comparison Worksheet

Chapter 6

Hire to 3-Month Checklist

Orientation Calendar Guidelines

Chapter 7

Partnership Protocol Snapshot Self-Assessment

Performance Platform Reminder Card

Chapter 8

Vision & Values Worksheet

SHIFT Reminder Card

Department Brand Exercise

Chapter 9

One-on-One Meeting Template

Staff Meeting Agenda

E-mail Rules of Thumb

DATA Driven Discussion Reminder Card

Chapter 11

Team Survey

Meet & Greet Cheat Sheet

Chapter 12

PIE in the Sky Exercise

Conference Attendance Application

Chapter 13

Stress Reduction Meeting With Your Boss

Book Group Guide

,

Chapter 14

Resignation Checklist

Chapter 15

Termination Meeting Checklist

If you have a great form that you use, and you want to help other nurse managers save time, email it to me at vicki@vickihess. com and I'll post it on the site for others to access.

REFERENCES

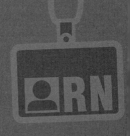

American Association of Critical-Care Nurses. (2005). *Standards for establishing and sustaining healthy work environments.* Aliso Viejo, CA: AACN. 1-9.

American Nurses Association. The nursing process: A common thread amongst all nurses. (2010). Retrieved from http://www.nursingworld.org/EspeciallyForYou/StudentNurses/Thenursingprocess.aspx

American Nurses Credentialing Center. (2009). Retrieved from http://www.nursecredentialing.org

Babcock, P. (2008). Watch out for the minefield of hidden bias. *SHRM Supervisory Newsletter.* Retrieved from http://www.shrm.org

Beebe, S., & Masterson, J. (2003). *Communicating in small groups: Principles and practice* (7th ed.). Boston, MA: Allyn & Bacon.

Bernthal, P., Rodgers, R.W., & Smith, A. (2003). Managing performance: Building accountability for organizational success. *DDI Executive Summary*, 1-5.

Blessing White. (2005). 2005 Employee engagement report. Princeton, NJ.

Blessing White. (2008). 2008 Employee engagement report. Princeton, NJ.

Buckingham, M., & Clifton, D. (2001). *Now, discover your talents.* New York, NY: Free Press.

Childrens Hospital Los Angeles. (2009). Our mission & vision. Retrieved from http://www.chla.org/site/c.ipINKTOAJsG/ b.3579013/k.9407/Mission__Vision.htm

Corporate Leadership Council. (2004). Employee engagement survey. Retrieved from https://clc.executiveboard.com/Public/ Default.aspx

Crandell, S. (2009). The two lenses of talent management. Retrieved from http://www.talentmgt.com/performance_ management/2009/October/1085

Eastern Kentucky University. Performance management guide. (2007). Retrieved from http://www.hr.eku.edu/development/ performance/resources.php#rating

Falcone, P. (2002). *The hiring & firing question and answer book*. New York: AMACOM.

Falcone, P. (2009). *101 tough conversations to have with employees*. New York: AMACOM.

Heathfield, S. (n.d.). Discipline (progressive discipline). About. com. Retrieved from http://humanresources.about.com/od/ glossaryd/a/discipline.htm

Hess, V. (2008). *SHIFT to professional paradise: 5 steps to less stress, more energy & remarkable results at work*. Dallas, TX: CornerStone Leadership Institute.

Hewitt Associates. Engagement and culture: Engaging talent in turbulent times. (2009). Retrieved from http://www.hewittas- sociates.com/_MetaBasicCMAssetCache_/Assets/Articles/209/ hewitt_pov_engagement_and_culture.pdf

Hotko, B. Rounding for outcomes. *Hardwired, 1*(1). Retrieved from http://www.studergroup.com/newsletter/Vol1_Issue1/ roundingforoutcomes.htm (2004).

Johnson, R. (2007). What's new in pedagogy research? *American Music Teacher, 57*(2), 58-60.

Lawyers.com. (n.d.). Employer: At will employment FAQ. Retrieved from http://labor-employment-law.lawyers.com/employment-contracts/Employer-At-Will-Employment-FAQ.html

Leaf, M.J. (2005). The message is the medium: Language, culture, and informatics. *Cybernetics & Systems, 36*(8), 903-917.

Lencioni, P. (2002). *The five dysfunctions of a team: A leadership fable*. San Francisco, CA: Jossey-Bass.

Lockwood, N.R. (2009). Society for Human Resource Management. Retrieved from http://www.shrm.org/Pages/default.aspx

Noe, Raymond. (2009). *Employee training & development.* New York, NY: McGraw Hill/Irwin.

Paller, D.A., & Perkins, E. (2004). What's the key to providing quality healthcare? *Retrieved from http://gmj.gallup.com/content/14296/whats-key-providing-quality-healthcare.aspx*

Robinson, J. (2008). Turning around employee turnover. *Gallup Management Journal*. Retrieved from http://gmj.gallup.com/content/106912/Turning-Around-Your Turnover-Problem.aspx

Rodgers, R.W., Bernthal, P., & Smith, A. (2003). Managing performance: Building accountability for organizational success. Retrieved from http://www.ddiworld.com/pdf/ddi_performancemanagement_executivesummary_rr.pdf

Smart, G., & Street, R. (2008). *Who: The A method for hiring.* New York, NY: Ballantine Books.

Smith, S, & Mazin, R. (2004). *The HR answer book.* New York: AMACOM.

Society for Human Resource Management. (2008). Documenting disciplinary issues. Retrieved from http://www.shrm.org/ TemplatesTools/Samples/PowerPoints/Documents/2008%20 Documenting%20Disciplinary%20Issues.ppt#292,34,Summary

Society for Human Resource Management. (2008). I would like to give managers easy-to-remember and easy-to-follow rules for applying discipline. What do you suggest? Retrieved from http://www.shrm.org/TemplatesTools/hrqa/Pages/disciplinetips. aspx

Stanton, M.W. (2004). Hospital nurse staffing and quality of care. *Agency for Healthcare Research and Quality, 14*, 1-12.

State of Maryland Department of Labor, Licensing and Regulation Division of Unemployment Insurance. (2009). What you should know about unemployment insurance in Maryland. Retrieved from http://www.dllr.state.md.us/employment/clmtguide/

United States Equal Employment Opportunity Commission. (2010). Prohibited employment policies/practices. Retrieved from http://www.eeoc.gov/laws/practices/index.cfm

Vermont Nurses In Partnership. (2010). Mission/vision statement. Retrieved from http://www.vnip.org/about.html

Wagner, R., & Muller, G. (2009). Whom do you trust? Retrieved from http://gmj.gallup.com/content/123881/Whom-Trust.aspx

Wagner, R., & Muller, G. (2009). No fair! Retrieved from http:// gmj.gallup.com/content/122837/No-Fair.aspx

Wasserman, N. (2000). A closer look at behavior-based interview- ing. Retrieved from http://www.inc.com/articles/2000/03/17957. html

Waterman, R.H., & Peters, T.J. (1988). *In search of excellence.* New York, NY: Grand Central Publishing.

Yeung, R. (2008). *Successful interviewing and recruitment.* Philadelphia, PA: Kogan

INDEX

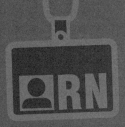